A WELLNESS GUIDE©

NATURES BENEFIT FROM CORAL CALCIUM

SECOND EDITION APRIL 2003

- SORTING FACTS FROM SPECULATION ON CORAL CALCIUM
- THE BENEFITS OF ONE OF NATURE'S MOST PRECIOUS SOURCES OF MINERALS AND CALCIUM
- CORAL CALCIUM IS NOT MERELY A "CALCIUM FACTOR" FOR HEALTH
- LEARN HOW EMERGING SCIENCE SHOWS THE HOLISTIC PROPERTIES OF CORAL MINERALS
- WHICH OF THE 100 OR MORE CORAL CALCIUM SUPPLEMENTS, IF ANY, SHOULD YOU USE?
- WHY CORAL CALCIUM IS NOT JUST A CALCIUM SUPPLEMENT
- DISPEL THE MYTHS AND POOR SCIENCE ABOUT CORAL CALCIUM
- UNDERSTAND THE CLAIMS ABOUT "FORMULAS "

By
Stephen Holt M.D.

www.naturesbenefit.com
www.wellnesspublishing.com
www.coralcalciuminformation.com
www.coralcalciummagazine.com

www.wellnesspublishing.com
www.coralcalciummagazine.com

Book cover design and typesetting by Asha Azhar and Jonathan Gullery.

Manufactured in the United States.
Library of Congress Cataloging-in-Publication Data.
Holt, Stephen 1950 –

Title: "Natures Benefit from Coral Calcium: A Definitive Guide".

ISBN – 0-9714224-4-3
SECOND EDITION

1. Coral 2. Health Benefits 3. Calcium 4. Coral Calcium 5. Minerals 6. Longevity 7. Alternative Medicine 8. Fossilized Coral 9. Coral Sand Collection 10. Coral Sand Processing 11. Nutritional Medicine 12. Dietary Supplements 13. Bruce Halstead 14. Robert Barefoot 15. Coral Calcium Powder 16. Coral Calcium Capsules 17. Dietary Supplements 18. Coral Sand Supply 19. Coral Reef Safety

A Note to the Reader:

The author of this book is not attempting to provide advice on the treatment or prevention of disease. While the health benefits of dietary supplements are reviewed, it is not the intention of the author to provide an alternative to the orthodox physician/patient relationship. Rather, it is the objective of the author to expand the dimensions of orthodox medicine by provoking more interest in remedies of natural origin. Food is being incorporated more into medical practices in the 21st century, where diet and lifestyle will play a dominant role in preventive medicine. This book was not written to endorse the use of specific products for any treatment purpose. The conclusions in this book represent the author's opinions of medical, scientific, folkloric and lay writings on the various topics discussed.

The publisher and author accept no responsibility for the use of any agents mentioned in this book. Before any individual self-medicates, he or she is advised to seek the advice of a qualified health care professional. The author does not support unsubstantiated claims of health benefits of foods or dietary supplements. This book must not be interpreted as product labeling.

www.wellnesspublishing.com

CONTENTS

FOREWORD

Coral Calcium has become one of the most popular dietary supplements in the history of the health food industry. Therefore, the importance of Dr. Stephen Holt's work must not be underestimated. Embroiled in controversy, coral calcium has been subject to material misrepresentation by many people who market and promote this dietary supplement. It is with great pleasure that I write this foreword to Dr. Holt's book which is a scholarly and balanced account of coral calcium and its potential biomedical significance.

I have had the pleasure to work closely with Dr. Holt and Natures Benefit Inc. in my capacity as a principal of Coral Inc. Dr. Holt has been described as an "icon" of the food and nutraceutical industry because of his many contributions to research, product development and education. I echo these comments, as Dr. Holt carefully sorts speculation from science in his approach to the subject of coral calcium.

The integrity of the author of this book shines through as it becomes clear that Dr. Holt resists the aphorisms of some marketing people who have been willing to say and do just about anything to increase their coral calcium profits. It is notable that Dr. Holt will not make premature judgments about the best type of coral calcium. He discusses the merits of high quality land and sea-based coral calcium, as he examines the facts on the subject. Nor does Dr. Holt buy in to the absurd and illegal treatment claims made about this valuable supplement. These claims have been made in the media by marketing "predators." For the first time in the literature, Dr. Holt examines the origins of coral calcium in Okinawa and he reveals his painstaking research on product specifications and both collection and manufacturing of the material used in coral calcium supplements. This book dispels many of the myths and fallacies of the subject of coral calcium that have contaminated our understanding of this holistic source of minerals, including but not limited to calcium.

Dr. Holt is to be commended for his evenhanded reporting on many controversial issues, some of which I would prefer to see portrayed differently. These issues include the environmental impacts of dredging the ocean floor and the question of whether or not high magnesium can be naturally occurring in coral. But overall, the book strives to fairly present both sides and for that the dietary supplement industry should all be thankful. It is important to note that Dr. Holt, as a medical doctor, will not completely embrace the naturopathic theory of pH balance of the body as a primary effect of coral supplementation. However, he does not discount all of the possibilities.

This book is a rapid update of Dr. Holt's first book on the subject of coral calcium. The need for this book is great, given the proliferation of so many brands of coral calcium. Dr. Holt selects his statements carefully and presents a series of factoids on the subject. These factoids permit an individual to rapidly reverse the current misinformation that may dominate some areas of the dietary supplement market, especially the Internet and "TV promotions".

It is clear that Dr. Holt wishes to focus on the important issues of the quality of the coral calcium in supplements. He is not side-tracked by the "bells and whistles" added to the various formulas of coral calcium. Additives to coral calcium are alleged to enhance the product. It is clear that no superior "formula" of coral calcium exists. The real issue is the careful selection of a coral supplement using "clean" high quality coral and a product formula free of hazardous materials. In this context, Dr. Holt reacts against the inclusion of significant quantities of potentially toxic substances, such as cesium added to coral calcium supplements.

While good grounds exist to criticize several individuals or companies that have misrepresented the subject of coral calcium, Dr. Holt resists the negative. Most impressive about this work is Dr. Holt's willingness to state the facts, even though he recognizes that some people want to believe in "miracle cures". If anyone "senses" a negative aspect on the subject of coral calcium in this book, they may be being told "what they do not want to hear." This situation is unfortunate, but necessary, as Dr. Holt goes into combat with the purveyors of false promises of "cures" from dietary supplements.

Andy Bowers
Coral Inc. Nevada, March, 2003

PREFACE

Let me brighten the horizon of the second edition of this book by stressing my belief that coral calcium is a valuable, rediscovered remedy of natural origin with potential to promote health and well-being. Coral calcium is a natural, holistic mineral supplement that supplies many elements or micronutrients (minerals) that are absolutely essential for the chemistry of life. In fact, the name "coral calcium" does not do justice to this remedy of natural origin. Coral remnants or coral calcium appear to have much more to do with general micro-mineral supply to the body, rather than being merely another source of calcium in our diet. In other words, I do not believe that the health-giving potential of coral calcium is limited to its content of calcium alone.

In this book, I examine potential homeopathic or therapeutic mechanisms of action of coral calcium, related to its fascinating micronutrient profile. The supplement "coral calcium" suffers from its own name, for it is much more than just calcium. Furthermore, it suffers from "promoters" who focus on the "calcium factor" alone and who may be in need of more than a few lessons in basic biochemistry and medical science.

Please read this book with optimism. It will give you some insight into how difficult it is to sort science or fact from speculations (or rhetoric) when it comes to potentially valuable dietary supplements. It is even more difficult to correct irrational beliefs that have been planted in consumers' minds by "crackpot" dialogue in the media. The nutraceutical revolution is now part of mainstream medicine and a much greater burden of scientific proof has to be placed on scientists involved in developing supplements, as well as on supplement purveyors. I hope this book will encourage people to select the right kind of coral calcium supplements, and I trust that it may dispel some of the myths and fallacies that have crept into the biomedical application of one of nature's greatest treasures—fossilized or remnant coral from the sea and land mass of the Ryukyus Islands of Okinawa, Japan.

Stephen Holt MD,
Newark, NJ, March 2003

CHAPTER 1:

THE FOUNDATIONS OF CORAL CALCIUM

SORTING THE FACTS FROM SPECULATION

Depending on your preference for surfing the Internet or reading popular literature, you will find descriptions of the dietary supplement, coral calcium from Okinawa, Japan as either a panacea "treatment" or a "scam." Switch on the TV and listen to illegal treatment claims about coral calcium, but please pause and examine the comical, commercial commentary. I believe that coral calcium is neither a medical panacea nor a scam. Coral calcium is a valuable and holistic, mineral supplement that poses many important issues. These issues range from discussions about our current mineral-depleted Western diet to concerns about the ecology and future of coral reefs.

In the second edition of this book, I avoid discussions or claims about the treatment benefits of coral calcium, but I present some emerging science from Japan. Treatment claims about coral calcium have become apparent in many other contexts and many of these claims are preposterous. Instead of disentangling all of the current nonsense, I take a hard look at the origin of this dietary supplement with a desire to dispel some of the myths and fallacies that have emerged in the description of this health-giving, natural resource.

THE BIOLOGY AND GEOLOGICAL ASSOCIATION OF MARINE CORAL

I am only a student of the biology of Marine Sciences, not an expert. A living coral polyp has a mouth and tentacles that allow it to live by filtering seawater and consuming plankton. The living polyp secretes minerals, principally calcium carbonate, to form a hard covering or exoskeleton. After the coral forms its stony house other coral polyps grow on the hard foundation. "Limey" (calcium-rich) secretions of algae help to join the framework of coral reefs together. This process creates coral reefs which are the largest structures on earth that are built by any living organism.

The distribution of coral in temperate oceans is quite uneven throughout the world. Much coral lives in underwater zones that are adjacent to aggregations of volcanoes or seismic activity. Underwater volcanic activity or the remnants of this activity produce a mineral-rich environment in the seawater in Okinawa, Japan in which coral lives. Thus, live coral often filters mineral-rich seawater. The change of climate under the sea or simple wave action causes natural breaks in coral reefs. The reefs often shed a sand-like material. This coral sand is supplemented by other natural processes such as deposits from other marine life or various geophysical occurrences.

Coral sand contains dead coral (fossilized) that covers the ocean floors around the reefs. However, coral sand contains other fossilized remnants of marine life and it is often mixed with plant material, organic matter and marine fossils, with fragments of shells and silica (sand). Coral remnants are swept several miles away from reefs and over thousands of years some form islands or land masses. It is this coral sand that is processed to make the dietary supplement, coral calcium. **Live coral is not used as the precursor of coral calcium dietary supplements.**

Oceanographers have warned of the peril that threatens the survival of coral reefs (see *National Geographic*, Vol. 195, No. 1, Jan., 1999). Therefore, the issue of the environmental significance of using coral calcium as a food supplement has more than piqued the interests of conservationists. To date, no evidence exists that the collection of fossilized stony coral minerals (above-ground coral sand) or coral sand from the seabed has caused any environmental damage. Although coral calcium has nothing to do with live coral, there is some residual concern about how underwater deposits of coral sand may be collected (www.coralcalciuminformation.com).

The living coral reefs of the world form a meeting point for many ocean dwellers. The reefs are a rendezvous for one quarter of all species of ocean organisms. The evolutionary epicenter of coral material having the most different species of coral exists in Southeast Asian seas, but coral material can be found in unlikely places. Fossilized coral deposits are found in the American Midwest, where it was deposited millions of years ago (e.g. Bighorn Mountains of Wyoming and Montana). Dead coral deposits (fossils) are ubiquitous on our planet.

EARTH-SCIENCE, GEOLOGY AND OCEANOGRAPHY

Coral reefs are formed from the secretions of living coral and certain algae. These secretions are calcareous, meaning that they are composed mainly of calcium carbonate. Although the outer skeletons of the coral are the major components of the reef, there are many other skeletons of small animals and plants within the reef's hard framework which is built primarily by the living coral polyps. The entire structure of a coral reef is formed also by limey (calcareous) secretions of algae. Just in the way that "coral calcium" is misnamed because it is more than just calcium, the term "coral reef" does not include all of the other living or fossilized matter within the reef structure.

Reef-forming coral grows best in seawater with an average temperature of 75 degrees Fahrenheit (25 degrees Celsius) and coral polyps cannot survive without adequate sunlight. These obligatory conditions for coral growth limit the depth of reef growth to about 150 feet (about 45 meters). Many coral reefs may form interesting circles or atolls where continuous or broken rings of coral tend to surround a central lake of water (lagoon).

The mechanism whereby atolls form was described by the famous naturalist Charles Darwin, who suggested that coral reefs tended to form on the perimeter of sinking volcanic islands. This theory has been confirmed by modern geological-drilling experiments where the foundations of atolls have been shown to be composed of volcanic rocks. This basic knowledge of coral reef formation is important because the rich micromineral environment of volcanic rocks and soils contribute indirectly to enrichment of the exoskeletons formed by coral.

CORAL SAND AND SEA-FLOOR SEDIMENTS

Coral remnants used in coral calcium supplements are either the processed coral sand collected from the ocean floor around the Ryukyus Islands of Okinawa, Japan, or those mined from land deposits of coral sand. In general, the sea floor is covered with complex sediments of varying thickness. On ocean floors, miles away from land masses, mud is the most common form of sediment. Coarser types of sediment tend to occur as sand that is deposited on the continental shelves, nearer to shore lines. Much of this sand was deposited on ancient beaches that formed during the Ice Age. These beaches were submerged after long-ago phases of global warming caused the sea level to rise. The deposition of sediment on the floor of the sea is far from a simple process. Around the islands of Okinawa, the sea-floor sediment is specially enriched by fallen particles from coral reefs.

It is clear that sea-floor sediments have multiple origins, but the origin of the sediment found around the Ryukyus Islands is derived mainly from living organisms (coral reefs and associated marine life). This type of sediment is called "biogenous" sediment (bio=life, genous=formed, i.e. formed from life). Modern science has recognized three different origins of sediments that cover the ocean floor. One type is called "lithogenous" (originating from rocks) and one is called "hydrogenous" (originating from water). Lithogenous and hydrogenous sediments make a small contribution to the sediment on the shallow sea floors around Okinawa. The bulk of this sediment is biogenous and largely derived from coral reef droppings. This sediment is the coral sand that is the precursor of the dietary supplement coral calcium.

Because coral sand from Okinawa is largely biogenous, it consists of debris that is of organic origin from marine life. Within coral sand are the remnants of coral skeletons, but they are mixed with shells and skeletons of other marine animals and plants. Thus, **not all coral sand is from coral itself and therefore, not all "coral calcium" is from coral**. I stress this lack of uniform composition of coral sand because it has obvious bearing on any attempts to explain the biological functions of the supplement, coral calcium. Coral calcium is not simply the exoskeletons of dead coral polyps and this knowledge confounds understanding.

The debris found in coral sand also contains the remains of minute organisms that live in sunlit water. These microscopic forms of life settle to the bottom of the shallow water around the Ryukyus Islands and they may cause "calcareous oozes." These oozes are composed principally of calcium carbonate which is also the principal constituent of the exoskeleton of live coral.

Calcareous oozes are found in seawaters that do and do not contain coral reefs; these types of sediment fall on at least one half of the global ocean floor. Deep ocean water contains much carbon dioxide and calcareous oozes are dissolved at the depths of the oceans. This does not occur in shallow waters, such as those around Okinawa, Japan, where the biogenous sediment retains its content of calcium and other metals or minerals.

There are other biogenous types of sediment found in the oceans of the world. These include silaceous oozes and phosphate-rich oozes. Phosphate-rich oozes originate from fish scales, bones and teeth, whereas silaceous oozes are derived from the skeletons of radiolarian and diatoms (single-celled organisms). Figure 1 illustrates the shapes of minute calcareous and silaceous deposits that are typical of biogenous sediments.

**LIVING CORAL IS NOT USED
IN CORAL CALCIUM SUPPLEMENTS**

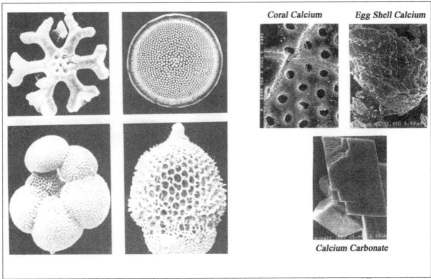

Figure 1A   Figure 1B

Figure 1A: High power microscopic examination shows calcareous and silaceous deposits that are derived from small marine animals and plants. Reproduced from data provided by the Deep Sea Drilling Project, Scripps Institution of Oceanography. These deposits form biogenous sediments and they complement the fragments of the exoskeleton of coral which is the principal component of coral sand. Coral sand is the precursor material that is processed to make the dietary supplement that is called "coral calcium". There are several reasons why the term coral calcium is a misnomer.

Figure 1B: High-powered microscopic photographs of coral calcium, egg shell calcium and calcium carbonate (plain). The porosity of coral calcium (43%) exceeds that of egg shell calcium and calcium carbonate. This enhanced porosity gives special physico-chemical characteristics to coral calcium. More minerals may dissolve when water is filtered through coral sand and more of the contents of the water may be extracted (loosely termed the "detoxifying action of coral sand").

Coral sand collected from the sea floor around the Ryukyus Islands of Okinawa varies in its mineral content. In certain locations the magnesium content of the coral sand is stated to be approximately 9% to 15% of the total mineral content (Marine-Bio Co. Ltd, Japan). The reasons why there are deposits of coral sand with high magnesium content is not completely understood and several suppliers of coral sand argue that this type of coral sand does not exist in a naturally occurring balance of calcium to magnesium of 2:1 ratio. Aggregations of coral sand may form with high magnesium content, in a similar manner to the development of manganese nodules that are found on the ocean floors in certain geographic locations distant from Okinawa. **The commercial suppliers of coral sand have a "raging argument" on the existence of a naturally, high magnesium content of coral sand.**

Coral calcium is a dietary supplement that is composed largely of coral skeletons and other retained fractions of biogenous sediments. This supplement is derived from remnants of living coral that have fallen from coral reefs, as a result of wave action or other natural processes. Over thousands of years, fossilized coral forms islands or mountains of coral. These deposits of coral can be harvested from land-based deposits, deep sea deposits and transitional zones that are tidal. As we start to address the location of coral deposits in Okinawa, even the distinction between ocean-derived and some types of land-based coral becomes unclear. Harvested coral can be treated by special processing techniques and then used as a mineral supplement in the diet. The word "fossil" implies that a dead organism is "antiquated" and can be "dug out" of the earth. I reiterate that I believe that all dead corals are fossils, so coral sand located underwater or above-sea level or at tidal interfaces is by definition "fossilized."

CORAL CALCIUM AND HEALTH: A MINI-ODYSSEY

It was the mid 1980s when I was introduced to the study of marine nutraceuticals by my mentors at Sun Yat-Sen University of Medical Sciences in Canton (Guangzhou), in the Peoples Republic of China. As a visiting Professor of Medicine at Sun Yat-Sen University, I was paired with my counterpart and close friend, Professor Liu (since deceased), who was the head of digestive diseases and nutrition at this prestigious university. In our private meetings, Professor Liu would "giggle" while relating fascinating stories about the Chinese Cultural Revolution. He interspersed his stories with his ideas about traditional Chinese medicines and other remedies of natural origin. His passion was to reveal his "health secrets" from the oceans.

As an allopathic physician with a strong belief in both pharmaceuticals and remedies of natural origin, I found it difficult to avoid expressing my skepticism to Professor Liu. As a true believer in Eastern medicines, he commented on the ability of nacre powder (oyster shell scrapings) to heal peptic ulcer and expressed his beliefs in coral grains (live coral and coral calcium) as a panacea treatment for all ills. Several years passed and my interest in marine nutraceuticals waxed and waned, but I became aware of increasing reports in the scientific literature about the power of several health products derived from the sea.

Despite my growing interests in ocean-derived medical remedies, I did not get excited in the "story" of coral calcium for health. The overriding factors causing my skepticism were the anecdotal descriptions of "panacea" benefits as a consequence of its use. When panacea claims for the health benefits of any supplement are made, one becomes naturally skeptical. Furthermore, I perceived the notable absence of hard-scientific data on the use of coral calcium as a remedy; and I had a stubborn disbelief that stony coral remnants could have many biological effects—they just seemed so inert. My mind started to change when I spoke with hundreds of individuals who had used coral calcium and claimed, in earnest, that they had experienced consistent health benefits.

In the mid 1990s, I had read about the drinking of water treated with teabag-enclosed coral and its beneficial health effects. The habit of drinking coral calcium-treated water was promoted initially by Scandinavians. My interest in coral was clinched when I watched a videotape interview of Erik Enby MD, a Swedish physician, who related his long-term experiences with coral treatments. My mind remained somewhat boggled by lack of explanations of how coral calcium could exert a health benefit. I did not embrace Dr. Enby's theories about coral minerals causing consistent and significant degrees of body alkalinity, but I could not disregard his anecdotal descriptions of described benefits with its use in many patients with different diseases.

My attention became directed to the work on coral calcium performed by the late marine biomedical expert, Bruce Halstead MD. This physician wrote a fascinating book about the health benefits of fossilized stony coral entitled, *Fossil Stony Coral Minerals and their Nutritional Applications* (available at www.wellnesspublishing.com). Unfortunately, Dr. Halstead died in November 2002, but I had a chance to interview him at length on the subject of coral calcium; information from this interview is contained in this book. In addition, I found some ancillary information about coral calcium-treated water and health in a booklet entitled, *"Why Calcium"?* Written by Dr. B. Owen (Health Digest Books, Cannon Beach, Oregon). Furthermore, a recent book, *"Calcium: The Facts"*, written by Beth Ley PhD, provides some anecdotes on coral calcium as a dietary supplement.

With growing enthusiasm about the supplement coral calcium, I collaborated with experts on the subject of coral calcium. I introduced several people, including Mr. Robert Barefoot, to different sources of coral sand. These types of coral calcium included the below-sea-collected, allegedly natural, calcium-and-magnesium-balanced coral calcium which is described in some detail in this book. Much information is to be found in the book, *Barefoot on Coral Calcium, An Elixir of Life* (www.wellnesspublishing.com). Since the initial writing of Mr. Barefoot's book more information and observations have surfaced about marine coral minerals. (The subject of coral calcium and health has been somewhat confused by Mr. Barefoot's inclusion of information on coral calcium in two of his earlier self-published books, *The Calcium Factor* and *Death by Diet*. This is an infringement of copyright held by Wellness Publishing.)

I have formulated dietary supplements associated with the likeness of Mr. Barefoot and Dr. Halstead. I attempted to form a series of holistic mineral supplements. Mr. Barefoot had proclaimed that "all coral (referring to all types of coral calcium) is fantastic." Dr. Halstead felt strongly that fossilized stony coral minerals (coral calcium), collected from ground deposits of coral sand, are the forms of coral calcium with the most advantages. The rest is contemporary history. The interest in coral calcium has swept the nation.

That said, I emphasize that I do not subscribe to several prevailing opinions on the best type of coral and, in particular, I do not support illegal treatment claims about dietary supplements. There is no doubt that illegal claims about the putative, curative properties of coral calcium have been made in the media, largely by predatory promoters of supplements and books that contain misappropriated copyright.

I stress that there are many people with interest in coral calcium and there are even more opinions on its value, or lack thereof. The frenetic interest in coral calcium and anecdotal claims of health benefits, which sometimes defy clear substantiation, prompted me to write and rapidly update this short book into a second edition. It is not my intention to give a fixed opinion on the biological significance of coral calcium or stony coral minerals, because there are many unknown issues concerning coral calcium. That said, it is time to dispel some of the myths and fallacies about coral calcium or stony coral minerals.

Coral calcium and all forms of coral minerals constitute a valuable category of nutritional supplements (regardless of whether they are derived from coral sand collected beneath or above-sea level). I will now dig a bit deeper and further attempt to sort some of the facts about coral calcium from the speculation. One may agree that speculation can be misleading.

CHAPTER SUMMARY

Coral calcium is misnamed. This dietary supplement is a holistic source of minerals, most notably calcium. The precursor material used to make coral calcium supplements is coral sand which is more than just the exoskeletons of dead coral. Coral sand is a biogenous sediment that can be collected below or from "washed-up" sources, above sea level. Preposterous treatment claims have been made about coral calcium. This may ultimately damage this valuable category of dietary supplements.

CHAPTER 2:

DEFINING CORAL CALCIUM SUPPLEMENTS: ORIGINS AND USES

DEFINING CORAL CALCIUM

Coral calcium from Okinawa, Japan is a holistic mixture of minerals in variable amounts. In general, the main elements found in fossilized coral or coral calcium are calcium and magnesium, but it also contains up to 70 or so trace elements, often in parts per million. Coral calcium in its fossilized form is best called "marine coral minerals" (a trademark of Natures Benefit Inc.) or perhaps "stony coral minerals". The term "marine coral minerals" refers to the fact that both ocean and land-based coral material are examples of fossils which are derived originally from a marine environment. Dr. Halstead (the revered marine scientist) objected to the terms "marine coral minerals" or "coral calcium" and he preferred to use the terms "fossilized stony coral minerals." Thus, the whole notion (or semantics) of what a fossil actually is has contaminated understanding about coral calcium. Furthermore, there is no evidence that one type of fossilized coral (collected beneath or above-sea level) exerts more measurable health benefits than another, despite the rhetoric (marketing nonsense).

At the outset, I wish to indicate strongly that coral calcium suffers from its own name. **Naming fossilized coral minerals as "coral calcium" has resulted in considerable confusion among consumers.** This situation has caused healthcare consumers to focus their thoughts inappropriately on calcium alone as they consider the nutritional value of coral calcium (marine coral minerals or fossilized stony coral minerals). Furthermore, this misconception has opened the door of criticism from individuals who describe inappropriately the disadvantages of coral calcium as "merely" a calcium supplement.

Some misguided individuals have contributed to this confusion by stressing "The Calcium Factor," a title of one book that expresses some incomplete and inaccurate information and misguided opinions on the biological role of calcium in the diet and related issues (www.quackwatch.org). The book, *The Calcium Factor*, bears the name of the late Carl Reich MD, but it has been revised several times since his death. I believe that the promotion of a book focusing on the element calcium in coral calcium (and claiming it to be the key active component of coral calcium) has led to consumer confusion and minimized the potential value of a complex nutraceutical. Dr. Reich had never made any documented statements about coral calcium as a supplement prior to his death, according to Dr. Bob Owen who has many of Dr. Reich's original writings in his possession.

ABOVE- AND BELOW-SEA CORAL CALCIUM ARE BOTH BENEFICIAL

The late Bruce Halstead MD, a marine expert and physician, had focused his work on the benefits of fossilized stony coral collected above ground, whereas others, including myself, have regarded *all* coral sand as being potentially health-giving, at least as a holistic source of minerals. Mr. Robert Barefoot, the arch promoter of coral calcium, is quoted repeatedly as saying that "all coral is fantastic", but it is hard to define where his loyalties lie with different forms of coral calcium.

Mr. Barefoot has endorsed and promoted the use of water treated with teabag-enclosed coral calcium, fossilized minerals collected above the sea level and below-sea collected coral, with varying opinion over time. More recently, he has developed an affinity for extolling the advantages of below-sea coral, but has not presented clear evidence that it is clinically superior to other forms of coral, despite his assertions. Mr. Barefoot has loaned his likeness to many different forms (formulae and types of coral calcium) of coral calcium supplements. Television infomercial companies that use separate interviews with Mr. Barefoot to promote their coral calcium products sell both above-ground-collected and below-sea level collected coral of varying types in varying formulations. This has confused consumers, some of whom have responded by believing the illegal treatment claims made in the TV infomercials.

Upon careful review, I can find no credible evidence whatsoever that one form of high-quality coral—collected above or below-sea level is superior or inferior to other forms, despite unsubstantiated claims to the contrary. In fact, emerging science that is discussed in Chapter 6 suggests relative advantages for high-magnesium and low-magnesium forms of coral calcium; including those found below-sea level (or adjusted by magnesium addition during manufacturing) and lower-magnesium containing coral calcium, found typically in land deposits. There are many characteristics of coral sand that determine its suitability for use as a food or dietary supplement. These include its mineral contents, mode of processing and a consideration of the collection process, used to obtain the coral sand, with special consideration for techniques that will not damage the environment.

There is much variation in coral calcium supplements and some companies sell coral calcium that is cut with plain calcium carbonate (chalk). When coral is used as a food supplement in human nutrition, the avoidance of contaminants in coral calcium (especially ocean pollutants) is very important. Heavy metal contaminants seem to be more common in unprocessed or poorly processed "deep" sea-collected coral. In fact, Dr. Halstead's biggest concern about coral sand collected beneath sea level is its *potential* content of pollutants, such as plutonium. This concern seems to be unfounded as careful tests on certain coral supplements show no evidence of such contamination and no evidence of dangerous levels of radioactivity (www.naturesbenefit.com).

Most forms of coral sand used in coral calcium supplements are not polluted by radioactivity or chemical pollutants. These opinions are debated by many interested parties; and the protagonists of below-sea coral argue that organic chemical pollutants are more likely to occur in land-based coral sand, but I find little evidence to support this opinion. One may see how the subject of coral calcium is cloaked in rhetoric and argument.

HOW STONY CORAL FORMS

There are two basic types of living coral, "soft" and "hard-stony" coral, both of which belong to the same general category of organisms as jellyfish, hydroids and sea anemones. It is the stony type of coral that forms a hard outer covering of minerals (exoskeleton). The elaboration of this outer skeleton by coral polyps (which are soft) takes many years; this process occurs as a consequence of the living coral polyp extracting food and minerals from sea-water. Thus, **the contents of coral calcium contain most minerals present in seawater**, which in turn contains most elements or salts available in the earth's crust (including perhaps in <u>some</u> cases, some modern industrial pollutants). Unfortunately, the coral and other marine organisms will tend to concentrate pollutants from the environment such as heavy metals (e.g. mercury, lead and cadmium) or organic chemicals, e.g. PCB's (polychlorinated organic compounds). That said, coral calcium is available for use in dietary supplements in forms that are free of any significant amounts of such pollutants (www.naturesbenefit.com).

All sea dwellers have an unfortunate tendency to be at the mercy of environmental pollution. The issue of toxic compounds in seafood has become a major public health concern, especially in waters abutting mainland Japan. However, the waters around Okinawa are considered to be quite clean. One must be aware that severe illness from heavy metal contamination (e.g. mercury poisoning) has been recorded close to industrial zones in several Eastern Asian locations, especially in mainland Japan. For these reasons, a discussion of sources and types of processing of coral remnants is particularly relevant (see www.naturesbenefit.com). Furthermore, these issues are of great relevance to the ecology. Coral reefs are threatened and any collection process that threatens survival of the coral reefs must be avoided (www.coralcalciuminformation.com).

Coral reefs are a very important focus of marine life. I reiterate that at any one time, a large proportion of sea-dwelling organisms visit temperate waters where coral reefs are found; and the coral reefs have their own rich array of inhabitants. With the popularization of coral calcium as a food supplement and increasing pressure to harvest coral remnants from the sea (and from land adjacent to water), the issue of environmental protection for the Ryukyus Islands must become a concern. Fortunately, the environment in Okinawa has been well-policed by the Japanese Government. At present, no damage to coral reefs around Okinawa, Japan has been observed or reported, despite increased collection of coral sand. These matters are discussed in greater detail in later sections of this book.

COLLECTION AND PROCESSING OF CORAL SAND

I have interviewed and corresponded with many suppliers of bulk coral calcium material from Okinawa, Japan. Requests that I made for information about coral collection, coral processing techniques and measured compositions of various commercial forms of coral calcium products (marine coral minerals or fossilized stony coral minerals) have been <u>variably</u> answered. It is notable that many suppliers and distributors of coral calcium or "bulk" coral sand material have entered the U.S. market in 2002. This is a direct consequence of the recent success of this dietary supplement category. While there appear to be many types of commercially available coral calcium from Okinawa, these different types of commercial coral calcium or sand seem to be a product of the number of different companies supplying coral, rather than of different sources of the base materials of the crude coral remnants (the "coral sand"). These important coral remnants (coral sand or coral calcium) are used to produce the finished coral calcium, a dietary supplement.

The commercial production of coral calcium involves several well-kept secrets; the "coral processors closely guard their business operations. This circumstance has arisen largely because coral calcium is now a valuable commodity which is at the root of a competitive business environment, especially in the U.S. It is notable that much coral sand has been used as filler in cement in the Japanese construction industry. I am particularly grateful to the staff of Marine Bio Co. Ltd. of Japan who have been very forthcoming with information. Marine Bio has made a firm commitment to research the biological activity of coral and it is the leading corporation in the supply of coral calcium bulk material, as is Coral Inc. of Nevada, USA.

The Japanese government has taken steps to regulate the

harvesting of coral which comes from two basic sources. The first source is land-based collection (mining) and the second is sea- based collection (suction collections from ocean beds) using "big-pipes".

WHY FAVOR CORAL CALCIUM FROM OKINAWA, JAPAN?

Fossilized coral is found on many coral islands, but the geographic location of coral calcium with the most reported health benefits is Okinawa, Japan. Okinawa is a prefecture (province) in Japan, composed of a chain of coral islands (the Ryukyus Islands). Folklore, anecdotes and scientific literature describe coral from Okinawa, Japan to be health-giving.

Why Okinawan coral calcium has been favored over other types of coral may be more related to folklore than science. The associations of coral with the robust health and longevity in the Okinawan population are impossible to link causally. Several scientists (especially the proclaimed "Quackbusters") have argued that health and longevity in Okinawa, Japan can only be linked to coral calcium by coincidence. It could be argued that coral sand from other locations in the world may be health-giving as a mineral dietary supplement, but this has not been explored. However, there are commercial sources of bulk coral sand from places other than Okinawa that may be used in some dietary supplements sold in the U.S. (caveat emptor).

Some "researchers" have made the absurd proposal that living microorganisms in coral supplements are responsible for its health benefits. Even more preposterous are suggestions that the "microbes" are living in coral that is eaten as a food supplement and that these "living bacteria" exert a favorable effect on the ecology and function of the human gastrointestinal tract. Most people have learned that coral calcium is processed by methods of "strict" sterilization, often using heat or ozone to render the coral remnants "free" of bacteria and other microorganisms. Further, some undesirable processing techniques may involve heating coral to very "high" temperatures, to eradicate heavy metals which are contaminants in some coral, e.g. lead, mercury and organic chemicals (environmental pollutants).

The lines of popular reasoning about the health benefits of Okinawan coral go something like this: Okinawans live long in relatively good health. Their environment is mineral-rich as a consequence of the presence of coral. Mineral-enriched environments have been associated with longevity, e.g. mountain populations in Tibet and Northern Pakistan. Therefore, coral is the reason for longevity among Okinawans. While plausible at first sight, this reasoning has to be questioned (see Chapter 6).

While it is true that Okinawans live longer, on average, than mainland Japanese inhabitants, their lifestyle and diet differ substantially from other populations. Therefore, factors other than coral calcium may promote health and longevity in Okinawans. While mineral enrichment of several environments has been associated with longevity (Walford, 1986), excessive amounts of specific metals can cause disease. Although other factors operate in the health and well-being of Okinawans, coral calcium remains an interesting candidate as an apparent environmental contribution to good health in Okinawa.

In the book, Calcium: The Facts, Beth M. Ley PhD reports that fossilized coral calcium was first discovered in 1979. She described a 1979 interview by a journalist from The Guinness Book of Records with a gentleman in Okinawa who was, at that time, the world's oldest person.

Without references, Dr. Ley describes the findings of a team of researchers who concluded that the secret to the longevity of Okinawans was the drinking water, which contained large amounts of dissolved or suspended minerals. It is noted that when it rains in Okinawa coral deposits on the mainland are eroded and drinking water becomes milky due to its coral calcium content. Some people in Okinawa may drink this min-

eral-enriched water which has been referred to as "milk of the oceans." The association of several mineral-enriched environments with longevity is used by Dr. Ley (and others) to propose that the drinking of this minerals-rich water may contribute to the extended life of Okinawans. These opinions are arguable among some scientists, form hypotheses for others, but they are believed by many people. I believe that mineral-rich (hard) water is healthy.

Finding and studying populations with longevity (long life and good health) has fascinated medical scientists and anthropologists, who believe they will find the secrets of long life. Despite many attempts to find the "fountain of youth", the discovery of such an "elixir of life" has eluded all who have sought it.

Modern concepts of aging now stress the importance of healthy lifestyle as a key anti-aging factor (www.antiagingmethods.com). The lifestyle of the relaxed Okinawans may be very different from that of the urban Japanese. There are many differences in dietary habits, stress levels, exercise, and social habits that can be distinguished between the island dwellers (e.g. Okinawans) and urbanites. These lifestyle factors may operate variably to determine longevity or premature death. For these reasons, it may be very difficult to define the health-giving role of a single environmental agent, such as coral sand or coral calcium (marine coral minerals or fossilized stony coral minerals).

INFORMED OPINION ON CORAL SAND COLLECTION AND HANDLING

I have had the pleasure to conduct detailed interviews with several executives from the companies that collect, process and/or supply bulk coral calcium and sell branded products. The information obtained from several sources has complemented my own direct research with Okinawan suppliers of coral material. My colleagues have visited many coral processing facilities in Okinawa during the past two years and I have studied many available specifications of commercial forms of coral calcium and its precursor coral sands. In addition, I have directed independent laboratory analyses on finished coral calcium supplements. However, there are some companies in Japan with exclusive supply arrangements that do not discuss their operations in an open manner. Consumers should avoid coral calcium supplements where full disclosure in the source of the product is avoided (www.coralcalciuminformation.com).

There are companies that supply coral sand products only (collection operations), some that process it and many more that broker or sell finished coral calcium remnants, in Japan and the USA. Each company has variable support from research scientists and variable frequency of analyses of each coral product batch. There appears to be some inconsistency in processing and some other production matters are hard to define.

Contrary to other uninformed assertions, underwater types of coral sand are collected a long distance (more than one kilometer) away from the actual reef, using an underwater suction apparatus that is akin to a giant "Hoover". Some observers believe that the collection process disturbs the seabed as well as much of the underwater plant material. Again, others disagree. In order to address this issue of protection to the coral reefs, I asked Mr. Someya and his staff at Marine Bio Co Ltd to research the matters on my behalf.

The scientists at Marine Bio Co. Ltd. in Japan worked with Professor Tamotsu Oomori of the Department of Chemistry, Biology and Marine Science at the University of Ryukyus. Professor Oomari issued the following statement based on his research on November 29th, 2002:

> The coral grains that have been used by Marine Bio Co., Ltd., is weathered remains of fragments or debris of coral reef marine organisms such as living coral and other carbonate shells. These particles are originally formed in coral reef areas, sorted and weathered by tide and wave motions and/or by interaction with seawater. They accumulate at the sea bottom near the coral reef area where the current is gentle.
> The harvest of coral grain does not damage living coral,

but only naturally formed coral grains are collected. As, metaphorically speaking, with trees and leaves, we do not cut down the tree nor living leaves, but only gather the fallen leaves.

It is important to say that, as a regal subject, harvest of these grains is controlled under the Okinawa Prefecture Government regulation. It is considered that controlled harvest with a fully supervised environmental conservation does not harm the natural environment nor cause the exhaustion of reef-building coral grains.

According to a study by oceanographers, the annual production rate of the coral grains is estimated to be approximately 3kg/m2 in coral-reef-sea around the Ryukyus Islands. Since the coral reef-building sea area in Okinawa Prefecture is approximately 800k m2, it is calculated that approximately 2.4 million tons of coral grain is naturally produced annually. We can safely claim that at least 1.2 million tons of the fossilized (weathered) reef-building, coral grain is naturally produced annually. Therefore, harvesting 100 tons monthly (1,200 tons annually) is equivalent to 0.01% of the coral grains annual production, and we can say that there is negligible impact on the ecological system of reef-building coral and the environment at the present state.

Tamotsu Oomori
Professor, Department of Chemistry, Biology and Marine Science, Faculty of Science, University of Ryukyus

It has been reported that coral remnants are removed from locations that may enhance the growth of coral reefs. Some individuals argue that coral sand chokes the reefs and stunts its growth. This is probably speculation. There appear to be no adverse ecological consequences of harvesting below-sea coral sand. Indeed, the Japanese Government and the producers assert that there are no environmental problems present or anticipated. I believe that they are correct in their current proposals. What may happen in the future remains to be seen. That said, it is important to present other peoples' opinions, but their opinions are arguable. These opinions are stated below:

> *"Clearing large areas of coral rubble would certainly impact reef ecosystems, not only because coral larvae settle on rubble (which is well-documented), but also because there are countless organisms that inhabit spaces within corals and rubble. Removing coral rubble from areas where the underlying sediment is unsuitable for larval settlement would certainly inhibit new corals from attaching and growing. I can't conceive that this practice would not negatively affect the long-term integrity of most coral reef ecosystems. There are other complexities, such as the removal of coral rubble that would change micro-flow patterns near the underlying substrate, in turn affecting the setting ability of coral larvae."*

> *Dr. Michael Dowgiallo, PhD*
> *Coral Reef Program Coordinator*
> *National Oceanic and Atmospheric Administration (supplied by Coral Inc, Nevada)*

> *"I would have an extremely hard time believing anyone who suggests that this activity would be benign. Dead corals may act as a substrate for new colonizers, so vacuuming up even dead corals or coral fragments might hinder the ability of reefs to recover in the future. Even if dredging/vacuuming is occurring where there are no (or few) corals, there are certainly other organisms being directly affected, such as sea whips and anemones, many of which also provide structure to benthic habitats and thus providing essential ecosystem functions (such as hiding places for juvenile fish and substrate for various life stages of benthic invertebrates)."*

> *John Clark Field, PhD Candidate*
> *School of Aquatic and Fisheries Sciences*
> *University of Washington*
> *(supplied by Coral Inc, Nevada)*

"This activity can harm the corals and the organisms that live in and on them in two ways. First, the dredging and vacuuming activity loosens and stirs up large amounts of sediment in the water. This sediment smothers and kills corals and other organisms in the ecosystem. An additional adverse effect of stirring up the sediment with dredging and vacuuming activities is that the turbidity of the water prevents light from reaching the corals, and the corals need light in order to survive and grow. Secondly, reefs are formed (and grow) by a process of bioaccretion (cementing together) of carbonate particles that have been removed from the living coral by bioerosion. If all the sediment that has accumulated around a reef (especially that which has already begun to solidify and hence does not risk smothering the reef) is scraped away, the reef loses its capability to grow and keep up with sea-level rise. Failure to grow and keep pace with sea-level rise would mean the demise of the reef because the corals need light and thus must be near the surface in order to live."

Mr. Majorie L. Reaka-Kudla, PhD, Professor,
Department of Biology
The University of Maryland (supplied by Coral Inc,
Nevada)

TYPES OF CORAL SAND AND ITS PROCESSING

The determination that there are two basic forms of "fossilized" coral, either land-based or sea-based, begets an obvious question: Which type is the best type?

Predictably, the answer to this question is not simple. I believe that both types of coral calcium are potentially health-giving. Unfortunately, many ill-informed opinions have been expressed on the best form of fossilized coral and this has caused massive confusion in the dietary supplement market, especially among consumers of potentially valuable coral calcium supplements. Contrary to popular misconceptions, the best type of coral sand material is not necessarily derived from ocean-based or land-based coral sand deposits. There are good and bad types of land-based and sea-based coral sand or coral remnants. The real answer to this question on the best types of coral is that each type may have different advantages and potential disadvantages, and appropriate selections must be made based on informed opinions (www.naturesbenefit.com, www.coralcalciuminformation.com).

The widely perceived advantage of below-sea collected coral has been related to its availability in a form with enhanced magnesium content, in comparison to the lower magnesium content of other ocean coral sand or land-based coral. In contrast, **land-based coral may have greater calcium content per weight than some below-sea coral**, at least in its finished format as coral calcium. Again, I stress that the health benefits of coral calcium (marine coral minerals or fossilized stony coral minerals) may be much more a function of its general mineral content—up to approximately 70 trace minerals or elements—than its content of calcium alone.

AVOID INFERIOR CORAL CALCIUM

While the word "inferior" describes some forms of land- or below sea level-collected coral sand, better words may be "potentially dangerous". Unprocessed, cruder forms of below-sea-collected coral sand may have a higher lead content, or toxic heavy metal content, than other forms of coral calcium. Furthermore, these types of coral calcium do not conform to certain U.S. government regulations, such as Proposition 65 in the State of California, an Act of Government designed, in part, to protect citizens against toxic factors in their environment. For these reasons, I restrict most of my statements on the use of coral calcium to forms of coral calcium supplements that are collected and processed in an appropriate manner (www.naturesbenefit.com).

My recommendations are based upon disclosures by manufacturers of coral calcium, concerning issues that determine safety. When it comes to purchasing a coral calcium supplement, the adage, *caveat emptor*, must apply. Beware discounted coral calcium! Some sellers of dietary supplements have labeled their products as containing coral calcium but they have combined small amounts of actual coral calcium with larger amounts of plain calcium carbonate. These products retail for less than $10 a bottle and sometimes up to $15. Well-processed, high-grade coral calcium is not cheap!

The form of below-sea collected coral that is safe and preferred is treated and screened for its heavy metal content, especially lead and mercury (www.naturesbenefit.com). This form of coral is available in different grain sizes (www.naturesbenefit.com). It is, predictably, an expensive form of coral and it is balanced with calcium and magnesium in a 2:1 ratio, by addition of magnesium or naturally occurring high magnesium content. I still find the proposal that a perfect balance of calcium to magnesium in a ratio of 2:1 exists naturally in coral sand to be doubtful.

As previously stated, marine coral has been preferred by some because of its "alleged" higher natural magnesium content. Elements may leach out of land-coral over years, but land-based coral can still be shown by analysis to contain trace elements. While I believe that elements can leach out of land-based coral, why would only magnesium leach? The professed advantage of the alleged, highest quality coral sand (collected underwater) is its apparent two-to-one balance of calcium to magnesium. Laboratory analysis of this type of "processed" marine coral (Sango Marine Product, SMP) shows variable calcium content (no less than 24%) with relatively high magnesium content (no less than 11%). This ratio is stated by the suppliers to be a natural occurrence in specific, but secret, locations in the waters around the Ryukyus Islands. Other suppliers argue with vehemence that this form of coral sand is not "naturally occurring."

ABSURD COMMENTS ON 'INFERIOR' FORMS OF CORAL CALCIUM

Some promoters of coral calcium supplements claim that other coral calcium supplements are "inferior" where the only quality of inferiority is a different "final presentation" of the supplement in the market in some arbitrary "formula". While contaminated coral calcium or coral calcium supplements that are cut with chalk (inorganic calcium carbonate) are inferior, nobody can say one form of high-quality coral calcium is inferior to the other, whether or not it is high or low in magnesium content or it is collected from the land mass of Okinawa or from the ocean floor around the islands of this province of Japan. The reader may note that "much" has been made out of the magnesium content of sand coral, but the evidence for the advantages of high magnesium content (an arguably better biological effect of coral calcium on the body) is still quite lacking.

Despite libelous statements made in advertisements about the inferior nature of land-collected coral calcium, there is no evidence whatsoever that land- or sea-collected coral sand is a better precursor for coral calcium supplements than the other. This libel (relating to statements about "profit" extortion) has attracted appropriate lawsuits or intentions to sue in the dietary supplement industry (see Chapter 7). In summary, our current level of scientific knowledge does not support the benefits of one form of high-grade coral calcium over the other (see Chapter 6).

BLENDED CORAL

While several people doubt the existence of "perfect" coral sand, as defined by naturally occurring 2:1 calcium to magnesium balance, I reiterate that the suppliers of this balanced coral calcium have stated that there is a specific location where this type of naturally occurring 2:1 calcium to magnesium-balanced coral sand exists. I have recently researched certification of this fact from suppliers and my earlier questions have been answered. In September 2002, I was sent samples and specifications on three lots of unprocessed coral sand which imply that this coral calcium precursor material has approximately 11% magnesium content. This high magnesium content is attributed by Marine Bio Co., Ltd. to be related to a specific, but secret, underwater collection point. Blending of coral calcium to increase its magnesium content is undertaken by manufacturers of coral calcium supplements. This practice is quite acceptable, but this type of coral calcium product is said to be different than the natural 2:1, calcium to magnesium ratio found in the coral supplied by Marine Bio Co., Ltd. What the difference "really is" is not clear.

It seems (according to some sources) that the below-sea coral used in supplements is created by a blend of coral material collected from the ocean floor using coral sand of variable magnesium content. I believe that this form (and other forms) of blended coral calcium is high-quality bioactive marine material that represents an excellent holistic source of minerals (see Emerging Science in Chapter 6). Highly recommended forms of below-sea collected coral sand exist in several dietary supplements (e.g. Barefoot Coral Calcium Plus™, Marine Coral Minerals™, Natures Benefit Inc. of Newark, NJ, www.naturesbenefit.com); as do high quality forms of land-collected coral (Halstead Coral Calcium™ and Coral Calcium Powder™, Natures Benefit Inc.).

CHAPTER SUMMARY

There is much to learn about the correct selection and handling of coral sand precursors that are used in coral calcium supplements. I reiterate, no evidence exists that land-collected coral sand are better than those collected below sea level, and vice versa. Much misinformation exists on which is the "best type" of coral calcium and the source of this information is often "marketing statements", not necessarily reality.

CHAPTER 3:

USING CORAL CALCIUM SUPPLEMENTS

THE IMPERFECT WORLD OF CORAL CALCIUM

By now, one can see that the world of coral sand collection and processing is not ideal and it is highly complex. Turning attention to land-based coral sand (mined), some individuals have made a case that this form may be highly desirable for use as a food or dietary supplement, at least in terms of its calcium content, and perhaps its significance to the environment. This opinion was espoused strongly by Bruce Halstead MD in his book on fossilized stony coral minerals. While Dr. Halstead commands a respected opinion given his background, training and contributions to marine medical science, there is no current evidence that collecting coral sand from the ocean floor around Okinawa is causing damage to the environment.

Land-based coral contains up to 40% calcium (35% - 37.5% in recent analyses), but its magnesium content is often less than 1%. Please note, the same applies to many types of marine coral calcium, especially those types used in "teabags". Consumers must recognize that much coral sand collected below sea level has similar low magnesium content to above-sea-collected coral sand. The types of below-sea coral sand collected and processed for use by Natures Benefit Inc. in two of its coral calcium products differ (Barefoot Coral Calcium™ and Marine Coral Minerals™ sold in recommended doses of 1.5g/day) because of its final Ca: Mg, 2:1 balance, during manufacture or supply. A lower content of magnesium in some forms of high quality coral calcium can easily be compensated for by adding a suitable magnesium source (e.g. magnesium oxide or carbonate).

It is argued that most published testimonials in the U.S. may have come from the use of land-based coral calcium in dietary supplements or even the use of water treated with coral enclosed in tea bags (some using land-based or below-sea collected coral sand in the tea bags). Therefore the issue—"Which is best, land- or below-sea-level coral material?"—remains the subject of debate and a lot of uninformed rhetoric (see Chapter 7). The claim that land-based coral sand is not a useful precursor of dietary supplements is merely marketing avarice and it is not an opinion supported by science. **Both forms of coral calcium, precursor material have been associated with claims of major health benefit, but many of these claims are anecdotes.** Table 1 summarizes some of the issues (matters of fact) related to different types of coral.

Below-Sea Coral Calcium	Land-Based Coral Calcium
Some types relatively low in calcium	Up to 38% calcium, +/- 10%
Higher magnesium (natural, added or blended?)	Magnesium easily and appropriately added, but not definitely required?
Ecological concern, but no damage reported.	Less concern about environmental consequences
More heavy metals and other sea pollutants in untreated forms?	Less toxic metal contamination, but more chemical pollution?
Processed with heat	Processed often with ozone, sometimes with heat
Health benefits described (anecdotal)	Health benefits described (anecdotal)

Table 1: Exploring some of the pros and cons of marine and land-based coral calcium. Note, both types have been used in capsules, powders and teabags. I believe that both types of coral sand may be useful as coral calcium supplement precursors.

OPTIMIZING CORAL CALCIUM USE

More important than discussions about sources and processing of coral calcium from Okinawa, Japan, are questions relating to the beneficial outcome of taking specific forms of coral calcium. These issues become nebulous when different types of coral calcium supplements are considered. There are few scientific studies of their use as nutritional "treatments" and testimonials of benefit, used to support the coral calcium product in question, do not always specify which kind of coral is being used by the reported beneficiary. In recent times, research has been undertaken on the biological effects of balanced below-sea coral (Ca: Mg, 2:1) and this research is reported in later sections of this book (see Chapter 6).

Many opposing opinions have surfaced to support the marketing of coral calcium supplements. In brief, Mr. Barefoot seems to prefer below-sea coral, but states confusingly that "all coral is fantastic." More confusing is his historic support for many different formats and types of coral calcium. In contrast, Dr. Halstead prefers land-based stony coral minerals for use in nutraceuticals (see www.naturesbenefit.com, for details of the products Halstead Coral Calcium™ and Coral Calcium Powder™). Dr. Beth Ley seems to lean towards the opinions of Dr. Bruce Halstead MD. I believe that the "jury remains out" on the "best" type of coral in the absence of comparative scientific studies.

There are varying sources of testimonials of health benefits, using below-sea and above-ground coral calcium taken in capsules, powders and in the form of coral calcium, teabag-treated water. I am personally aware of hundreds of people who have claimed benefit. While it is sometimes argued that testimonials are not absolute proof of benefit, one must be impressed by the sheer volume and consistency of supportive testimonials that have appeared in books, articles and "chat rooms" on the Internet. **Users of coral calcium are voting with dollars by re-ordering coral calcium supplements as a consequence of their perceived health benefits (www.naturesbenefit.com).**

A compilation of testimonials is present in Mr. Barefoot's book, *Barefoot on Coral Calcium: An Elixir of Life* (www.wellnesspublishing.com), but some of these testimonials may have been as a result of people taking coral calcium water derived from teabag-enclosed coral, some may be from the use of land-based coral and some allegedly from below-sea coral, at least according to some dietary supplement companies. This use of testimonials can be quite misleading.

CORAL CALCIUM IN THE DIETARY SUPPLEMENT MARKET

The dietary supplement industry is always encouraged when consumers show great excitement about a specific category of dietary supplements. Unfortunately, there is a less desirable segment of the industry that may broadcast misinformation and unproven claims about a dietary supplement. Such individuals are considered the arch enemies of the dietary supplement industry and recent history has confirmed this notion. Since the writing of my first edition of this book, there has been an explosion in the number of different brands of coral calcium available for sale. Each new brand tends to confound purchase decisions, sometimes as a consequence of misleading advertising.

Perhaps the most serious problem of all occurs when illegal treatment claims are made about a dietary supplement. In the case of coral calcium, claims have been made on national television that individuals may be able to "grow a new brain," "throw away their wheelchairs," and even "cure cancer." These are the tactics that give false promise to the desperate. The supplement industry must not support this form of predatory behavior, if it is to survive. I have had many unfortunate experiences of shattering some people's distorted beliefs about coral calcium after they have absorbed the absurd and preposterous treatment claims made by marketing predators. This situation has caused many people, including myself, much stress and anxiety.

I cannot claim to know everything about all forms of coral calcium that are being used in supplements, but I can report information that I know to be matter of fact. Only companies that have made careful independent analyses of the material that they both collect and use in coral calcium supplements should be supported in the "fragmented" dietary supplement market for coral calcium (www.coralcalciuminformation.com, www.coralcalcium-magazine.com). I report research information that was derived from studies by independent laboratories and, it is credible scientific data (see details in Chapters 5 and 6).

Specification sheets on coral calcium supplements and its precursor material (coral sand), have been exhibited by Natures Benefit Inc., Coral Inc., Marine Bio Co Ltd, and Optipure Inc. The derived specification sheets state mineral compositions that are only able to be verified in repeated testing. Independent analyses have shown predictable variations in the presence of macrominerals (calcium and magnesium) and microminerals (up to approximately 70 trace elements). Variability in composition of coral calcium and its sand precursors are present and expected. Coral sand found in the sea around Okinawa, Japan, is subject to variable conditions in seawater and marine life which have an obvious effect on altering the mineral composition of the coral remnants and other components of this "biogenous" sediment. Table 2A and Table 2B show the mineral profile of one type of balanced (Ca: Mg, 2:1) coral calcium (www.naturesbenefit.com).

COMPANIES WHO DISCLOSE THE MINERAL CONTENTS OF THE CORAL CALCIUM THAT THEY USE SHOULD BE SUPPORTED. ADDING CESIUM TO CORAL CALCIUM IS POTENTIALLY UNSAFE

(A) - Major Elements Found in Marine Coral Calcium

Assay	Per Cent(%)	PPM Metal
Silicon Dioxide	3.92	18,318
Aluminum Oxide	0.32	1,693
Calcium Oxide	33.60	240,000
Magnesium Oxide	18.90	114,000
Sodium Oxide	0.42	3,360
Strontium Oxide	0.33	2770
Iron Oxide	0.14	979
Loss on Ignition	41.30	
Total Majors	98.93	

NB: Loss on ignition occurs in the assay and it includes the total of water, carbon, nitrogen and sulfur

(B) - Trace Elements Found in Coral Calcium

	ppm		ppm		ppm		ppm
Al	1693	Hg	0.01	Mo	>1	Zn	16
Ag	7	La	2		(0.03mg)		(11mg)
As	trace	*Br	0.14	Nb	>1	Zr	>1
Ba	10	*D	150	Ni	7	*Os	>0.2
B	1	*Dy	0.18	P	280	*Pd	0.025
Bi	4	*Er	5.19		(700mg)	*Pt	>0.03
Cd	trace	*Eu	>0.1	K	830	*Pr	2.73
Co	11	*Gd	0.094		(2000mg)	*Re	>0.2
Cr	80	*Ga	0.692	Pb	trace	*Rh	>0.02
	(0.035mg)	*Ge	0.191	Rb	20	*Ru	0.081
Ce	20	*Au	>0.05	Sb	>2	*Sm	>0.05
Cu	23	*Ho	0.091	Se	14	*Sc	0.049
	(1.8mg)	*In	>0.06		(0.06mg)	*S	1780
Fe	979	*Ir	>0.04	Sr	2770	*Ta	>0.01
	(10mg)	*Li	0.66	Y	3	*Te	>0.02
I	9	Mn	20	V	20	*Sn	0.198
	(0.15mg)		(4.0mg)	W	0.1		
Hf	>1						

Tables 2A and 2B: Table 2A shows the major elements found in below sea-level collected, "balanced", coral calcium and Table 2B shows the trace elements. Data supplied by Natures Benefit Inc, NJ, USA with courtesy of Marine Bio Co Ltd, Japan, 2003. Note Calcium and Magnesium are present naturally as carbonate. The oxide measurements are the result of the measurement technique.

I believe that below-sea collected coral sand must be considered to be a fossilized form of coral calcium, just as above-sea level coral sand is composed of fossils. However, high magnesium containing types of coral calcium are not found in above-sea level coral sand. It is noted that coral sand is sterilized without alteration of the natural chemical contents of the coral sand (Table 2A and Table 2B). Few companies have actually shown that their finished product has a composition similar to the finished coral sand precursor (www.naturesbenefit.com). It is both the purity and selected size of the coral sand grains (micron size) that is often unique to high quality coral calcium products (www.coralcalciuminformation.com, www.naturesbenefit.com).

ANALYTIC TESTS OF CORAL CALCIUM

Later in this book, I describe a circumstance where the clinical benefits of different types of high-quality coral cannot be clearly defined, based on current levels of scientific knowledge. The balanced form of below-sea collected coral (Ca:Mg, 2:1) is the form of coral that has been subjected to recent scientific scrutiny. The independent testing on coral sand used for the production of dietary supplements is very valuable information. This scientific data has been acquired often by using state-of-the-art analytic technology (e.g. inductively coupled mass spectrometry). This type of analysis provides accurate measures of the minerals present in coral sand and coral calcium. These chemical analyses are able to detect elements in minute amounts (parts per million, ppm).

One of the main reasons for testing any coral calcium supplement precursors is to detect the presence of toxic heavy metals, especially lead and mercury. The presence of heavy metals are always a major concern when one examines new, natural mineral supplements or sources of calcium. While several forms of coral calcium do not contain excessive quantities of heavy metal such as lead or mercury, some may. Coral calcium formulae have emerged in the market containing milligram amounts of added cesium. Cesium has no biological role and it may be toxic. Consumers should support companies that sell coral calcium supplements with reported levels of heavy metals that are deemed safe and do not contain "high" added amounts of cesium (mg or greater) (www.natures benefit.com). Coral calcium supplements made with high quality, below-sea collected coral sand and some supplements containing selected types of above-sea coral calcium are free of significant levels of toxic heavy metals (www.naturesbenefit.com). These types of coral calcium conform to government legislation such as the "Safe Drinking Water and Toxic Enforcement Act" of 1986 in California, otherwise referred to as Proposition 65.

COMPARING CORAL SAND PRECURSORS AND CORAL CALCIUM SUPPLEMENTS

Responsible suppliers of coral calcium should be able to demonstrate that their coral calcium supplements have virtually the same composition as the crude coral sand that is collected from Okinawa, Japan. To my knowledge, the only type of coral sand that has been subject to this type of testing in a rigorous manner are among the coral calcium products sold in the U.S. by Natures Benefit Inc. (www.naturesbenefit.com).

In recent studies, scientists took coral calcium supplements from shelves in retail locations and tested them independently. These studies were focused on the best-selling brands of coral calcium owned by Natures Benefit Inc. of Newark, NJ. Scientists undertook their independent studies from random samples of the products made by Natures Benefit Inc. sold under the labels Barefoot Coral Calcium Plus™ and Marine Coral Minerals™ (bottles of 90s count). Duplicate analyses showed that the Natures Benefit products conformed to Proposition 65. Not only did the Natures Benefit products contain material that was accurately reflected on the supplement facts panel, but the composition of the coral calcium was substantially the same as bulk material produced and supplied in Okinawa, Japan. These encouraging results show the maintenance of good quality control from the inception of manufacturing and processing of bulk coral sand through to its delivery to the end-users (consumers) of coral calcium supplements. At the time of writing, no other forms of coral calcium have been examined in this way, in an independent manner (www.natures-benefit.com).

CORAL CALCIUM MUST BE FREE
OF ORGANIC POLLUTANTS

While the mineral composition of coral calcium is very important, there is a responsibility for suppliers of coral sand to test for the presence of harmful or dangerous chemicals, such as pesticides or industrial pollutants. There are standards for this type of testing that are widely accepted in medical science. These standards are often referred to as USP, which refers to the U.S. Pharmacopoeia and the European Pharmacopoeia. Natures Benefit Inc. has been the recipient of independent testing of types of coral calcium that they use in their supplements. In this series of tests, none of a range of 39 potentially harmful or dangerous pesticides or chemical residues were detected in the products sold under the labels Barefoot Coral Calcium Plus™ and Marine Coral Minerals™.

CORAL CALCIUM MUST BE FREE OF RADIOACTIVITY

Recently, several people have discussed some residual concerns about the possible presence of radioactive materials in coral calcium. It has been stated that the locations where coral sand is harvested could contain radioactivity, including radioactivity that may have remained in the oceans as a consequence of the detonation of atomic bombs. This concern is unjustified in the case of below sea-level collected materials used by Natures Benefit Inc. These coral sand materials have been analyzed carefully for radioactivity.

Tests were undertaken to detect gamma-emitting and "man-made" radiation, and none has been detected in the material used in Barefoot Coral Calcium Plus™ and Marine Coral Minerals™ (90 size count). Very small quantities of Uranium-238 are found in coral calcium, as a completely natural occurrence. This situation is present in several forms of "natural" calcium, including coral calcium. Testing for these minute quantities of Uranium in coral calcium samples has demonstrated levels of radioactivity in the expected normal range (i.e. background radiation levels). I stress that this minute amount of Uranium is a natural form of radioactive element in the earth's crust, to which everyone is normally exposed.

CORAL CALCIUM MUST BE FREE OF MICROORGANISMS

Any expressed concerns about the presence of yeast, mold and bacteria in coral calcium can be dispelled. Coral calcium used in products sold by Natures Benefit Inc. does not contain any dangerous yeasts, molds or bacteria. Coral calcium used in Barefoot Coral Calcium Plus™ and Marine Coral Minerals™ (www.natures-benefit.com) is food-grade material. The claims by some people that coral calcium contains microbes (bacteria) which play a useful role in supporting the digestive tract of humans are ridiculous (a Robert Barefoot aphorism). While the human digestive tract does variably contain friendly bacteria that promote general health (probiotic bacteria), coral calcium does not contain such bacteria. Infomercials have focused on the potential presence of such microbes and the statements made about this subject on TV are not supported by any reasonable scientific opinion.

CORAL CALCIUM IS WELL ABSORBED

Marketing companies continue to stress the good absorption of calcium into the body that can result from taking coral calcium as a supplement. While coral calcium is well absorbed, it is not "100%" absorbed, as falsely claimed. Experiments have been performed with the below sea- collected, balanced forms of coral calcium (Ca: Mg, 2:1) which show good absorption of calcium. Coral calcium contains calcium and magnesium that is combined with carbonate, but the minerals in coral calcium may be chelated (bio-inorganic binding), according to Dr. Bruce Halstead MD. The body does not utilize calcium and magnesium in the form of carbonate, and the chemical bonds must be broken by the body, in order that calcium and magnesium are able to exert their important biological functions within the body.

It is important to note that the forms of coral calcium used in Barefoot Coral Calcium Plus™ Marine Coral Minerals™, Halstead Coral Calcium™ and Coral Calcium Powder™ (www.naturesbenefit.com) can be ionized after the addition of acid simulated or gastric juice (stomach acid). Experiments showing this ionization of calcium in coral calcium have been performed in an independent laboratory, with the below-sea type of coral used by Natures Benefit Inc. Again, it is important for the non-scientist to understand that the demonstration of complete ionization of calcium in coral calcium in the laboratory does not necessarily mean that the calcium in coral calcium is 100% absorbed (this "alleged" 100% absorption is pure hype).

Experiments looking at the absorption of calcium from coral calcium in animals and humans show good calcium absorption (up to about 70%). I trust that it has become clear that biological benefits of coral calcium may not be solely related to its calcium or magnesium content. **Coral calcium is not a cost-effective source of calcium alone** and in the commonly recommended supplement dosages; it will not supply adequate recommended daily intakes of calcium for an adult. (except when taken as powder, see Natures Benefit, Coral Calcium Powder™). Some of the clinical benefits that occur with the use of coral calcium as a dietary supplement may be more related to its micronutrient profile (up to 70 or so trace elements), other than due to its content of calcium and magnesium alone. (See Chapter 5)

SOME COMPANIES LEAD THE WAY

Accepting that there <u>may</u> be some benefits to be derived from a higher magnesium content or a different micronutrient profile of below-sea coral fossils (arguable), a clear justification emerges for the use of both high-quality, below-sea collected coral calcium and high-quality, land-collected coral.

For these and other reasons stated earlier, Natures Benefit Inc. has created four different types of coral calcium supplements. Natures Benefit Inc. believes that it is important to define clearly the types of coral used in coral calcium dietary supplements. This need exists as the coral calcium category of dietary supplements expands rapidly. Natures Benefit Inc. has elected to use different forms of coral in its four products, based on available scientific data. Two of the products contain high-grade below-sea collected coral calcium (Barefoot Coral Calcium Plus™ and Marine Coral Minerals™). These products contain marine-collected coral in newly recommended daily doses of 1.5 grams per day in three capsules. The remaining two products contain land-collected coral calcium in a newly recommended daily dose of 1.5 grams per day in capsules (Halstead Coral Calcium™) or up to 3 grams per day in coral calcium powder (Coral Calcium Powder™). These latter two products are encapsulated fossilized, stony minerals called Halstead Coral Calcium™ (1.5g/day) or 100% Pure Coral Calcium Powder™ (3g per day) (see www.naturesbenefit.com). Unlike most other companies, Natures Benefit Inc. has published specifications of the constituents of its products with full disclosure.

DIET AND CORAL CALCIUM

Coral calcium is consumed in dietary supplements in the form of powders, capsules of different types (www.naturesbenefit.com) or by drinking coral calcium-treated water. Coral water is prepared most often by placing coral-enclosed teabags in drinking waters, but Natures Benefit Inc. has developed a convenient bottled version of alkaline-ionized water or coral calcium water (Coralyte™). Factors such as convenience, beliefs and nutritional intentions enter arguments about which is the best form of coral calcium product to take. Aside from these considerations, one must examine how coral calcium is used in traditional settings, such as those in Okinawa, Japan. Traditionally, coral calcium has been used as a certified food-grade supplement (Certified first in July 1989 by the Japanese Government) in a powder form for use in food preparation. For example, processed or fermented soy products such as tofu can be "set" during preparation by the addition of coral calcium powder. This firm "tofu" combines the health benefits of soy with calcium and mineral enrichment. **Calcium combined with soy protein has many potential health benefits including the nutritional support of bone health and cardiovascular health** (see Holt S., *The Soy Revolution*, Dell Publishing, Random House, 1999, available at www.wellnesspublishing.com).

Focused accounts of the health benefits of coral calcium for the citizens of Okinawa stress coral calcium as health-giving. I reiterate, however, that other factors operate to promote health in the population of Okinawa, Japan. The diet of the average Okinawan is very different from a Standard American Diet (SAD). The former is higher in fiber, essential fatty acids (omega-3), vegetable protein, fruit and vegetables and much lower in saturated fat, simple sugar and cholesterol intake than the latter. However, more salt may be present in the Okinawan diet–a negative issue that may be linked to the cause of increased problems with gastric cancer and stroke in Japanese people.

I have reviewed the role of soy in promoting health in Asian communities in my two books (Holt S, *Soya for Health*, Mary Ann Liebert Publishers Inc., Larchmont, NY, 1994; and Holt S, *The Soy Revolution*, Dell Publishing, Random House, NY, NY, 1999). The soy intake of Okinawans has peaked in recent years and it may be declining. I believe that soy in the diet of Okinawans contributes to their health and well-being. There is a tradition of eating pork in Okinawa often prepared in the regional dish called *champuru*, a stir fried dish of vegetables, tofu and pork. The dietary habits of Okinawans form the basis of some claims of relative good health and longevity that is present in these island dwellers.

HOW TO TAKE CORAL CALCIUM AS A SUPPLEMENT

It is logical to reason that "whole coral calcium" in powder or pills (below-sea level collected coral minerals or fossilized stony coral minerals from land masses) are the best ways to take coral calcium as a supplement. This may or may not be the case because credible scientists have linked the longevity and health of Okinawans to the drinking of coral water (see Coralyte™, www.naturesbenefit.com). Capsules or powders of coral calcium seem ideal and convenient when swallowed whole, added to food or taken by emptying capsules into beverages or to food. While I do not ignore that coral calcium water made from coral calcium-containing teabags has been associated with reported health benefits, coral calcium is relatively insoluble and **only a small percentage of the coral minerals dissolve in the coral water**. Thus, coral-treated water delivers only very small amounts of minerals and elements for absorption into the body. That said, there are alternative medicine concepts that described the benefits of small amounts of mineral intake (see the discussions of "cell salt therapy" and "lithiohomeopathy" in chapter 6)

The majority opinion on the best way to take coral calcium

is that it is best consumed in capsules with good dissolution characteristics. This mode of administration presents the "whole" coral calcium supplement for digestion and absorption in the gastrointestinal tract. **"New" coral calcium supplements have appeared as tablets (caplets) and soft gel capsules. The dissolution (release) of tablets or caplets of coral calcium has not been studied in a clinical context and there must be concern that the minerals in coral calcium caplets or tablets may not be well absorbed as they may be in capsules.** On the other hand, coral calcium-treated water could be homeopathic in its effects and a tendency to an extension of lifespan has been observed in laboratory animals that have been given alkaline-ionized water derived from water exposure to coral calcium.

Later in this book (Chapter 5), I discuss the "cell salt theory" or "Schuessler's Theory" of health maintenance (an extension of homeopathic medicine). These hypotheses may provide support for the use of coral water produced from exposure to coral calcium filtration systems or from teabag-enclosed coral. **The "cell salt theory" may be one mechanism whereby coral calcium exerts a health benefit.**

HOW MUCH CORAL SHOULD BE TAKEN?

The optimal daily dose of coral calcium (marine coral minerals or fossilized stony coral minerals) is a best guess. The answer to this question about the recommended daily intake of coral calcium is not only unknown, it is not simple. We have a confusing precedent upon which we can start to address the issue of ideal doses of coral calcium in supplements. First, the "traditional" use of coral calcium involves intake of at least gram amounts or greater daily, in food preparation. However, one may not dismiss the reports that coral water, containing only small amounts of dissolved coral minerals, may be beneficial for health. This enigma may be related to the knowledge that only small amounts of minerals (cell salts) may have beneficial effects (e.g. a homeopathic effect, or the "Schuessler effect"–see later). Homeopathy is a treatment science where infinitesimal amounts of various natural substances are believed to have treatment properties.

Anecdotally, good responses have been reported with daily

intakes of 1 gram (1000 mg of coral) of ocean-derived or land-based coral with or without the addition of magnesium. However, given the precedent for higher intakes of coral in traditional settings, I believe that at least 1.5 g. of coral calcium of either type (land- or sea-collected coral calcium), may be more optimal. My recommendations of at least 1.5 grams per day of coral calcium in three capsules are based on this reasoning. Higher doses of coral calcium are taken with convenience by the use of powders. The use of coral calcium powders in doses of 3g per day start to deliver the adult RDI (daily value) of calcium (greater than 1000mg of elemental calcium). Emerging science is clarifying the clinical effects of these higher doses (2.8 g per day) of coral calcium (see Chapter 6).

It has been argued that the higher the concentration of calcium taken from coral calcium the better, up to an *arbitrarily* recommended maximum of 2 grams per day of elemental calcium (levels greater than the RDI of calcium). I stress that calcium in higher amounts than recommended daily intakes (RDI) must be used only where they are indicated and known to be safe. Now comes an issue that may surprise the consumer. The current recommended daily amounts of intake of coral calcium by the majority of supplement companies do not even come close to meeting the current recommended daily intakes (RDI) of calcium that are considered by most nutritional scientists to be optimal. A little simple arithmetic (see below) will help to explain this important issue and reinforce my recommendation of increasing the amount of coral calcium intake to at least 1.5 grams per day (www.naturesbenefit.com).

CALCIUM CONTENT OF CORAL CALCIUM

High-quality, below-sea-collected coral contains about 24% - 38% calcium, so only 240 - 380 mg or more of elemental calcium is available from a dose of 1000 mg (1 g) of coral calcium. To supply a recommended daily intake of calcium of about 1000 mg (RDI 100% or less than RDI), one would have to take about 3g - 4 g of this type of marine coral. Average daily doses of coral calcium in most coral calcium products are recommended at 1000 mg in two capsules and to take the recommended daily intake (RDI) of calcium (assuming it to be 1000 mg per day) would require the taking of at least four "standard" coral calcium capsules! Even land-collected coral with its variably higher calcium content still does not meet the expectations of recommended daily intake (RDI) in dosages of coral calcium suggested by most manufacturers.

For these reasons, I stress that people who take coral calcium must still consider the importance of sticking with a calcium-rich diet or using other calcium supplements if necessary to achieve recommended daily intakes of calcium. The RDI of calcium for several groups of adults is set at 1200 mg per day of calcium. **I have found that the understanding of calcium intake with coral calcium is the single most confusing issue for consumers of coral calcium.**

On a practical level, I advise patients who are looking for optimal calcium intake (at the higher levels of RDI) to consume a diet that provides at least 500 mg of elemental calcium and try to supplement about 1000 mg of elemental calcium from other sources such as coral calcium, combined with other calcium supplements as necessary (see www.naturesbenefit.com, www.naturescalcium.com, www.antiporosis.com). These issues will become clearer as I discuss the general issues of calcium supplementation later in this book. That said, the focus on the "calcium factor" alone when it comes to coral calcium (a misnomer) is a limited and inaccurate perspective, produced by "promoters" of coral calcium.

OPTIMIZING THE CORAL CALCIUM SUPPLEMENT

Based on the information available and accepting its occasional limitations, my clear recommendations for an ideal coral calcium supplement emerge from the following:

- The calcium content of the coral may not be as important as hitherto supposed. In this respect, some types of land-based coral have been preferred over below-sea collected coral calcium; not only because of their relatively high calcium content but also because of their desirable micronutrient profile (many elements). Regardless of whether or not coral collected from above or below-sea level is used as a supplement, I see some advantages in adding extra sources of elemental calcium in the diet, if an RDI of 1000 mg (or greater) of calcium is desired (see Chapter 4, Section on Egg Shell Calcium or www.naturescalcium.com).
- Ocean-derived coral calcium has some putative advantages,

providing that high-quality, lead-free, pollutant-free coral is used (refer to land- and below-sea collected coral calcium, Barefoot Coral Calcium™, Halstead Coral Calcium Plus™, Coral Calcium Powder™ and Marine Coral Minerals™, www.naturesbenefit.com). Coral sand collected from the ocean floor or mined above sea level should only be used if it can be certified free of heavy metals or other contaminants (www.naturesbenefit.com). There is coral calcium available for use in supplements that may contain unacceptable levels of lead, and this form of coral is not approved for sale in the U.S., (refer to California State Legislation, Proposition 65 and see www.coralcalciuminformation.com).

- Coral calcium alone may not supply all required dietary calcium for most people in current common recommended daily intakes of 1g/day or greater. A dose of 1.5 grams per day of coral calcium is sometimes more desirable. Most marketed doses of coral calcium in supplements are probably too small (www.naturesbenefit.com).

- Nature's imprint for the correct assimilation of calcium by the body is believed by some to be calcium to magnesium balanced in a ratio of two parts calcium to one part magnesium. This is arguable. Benefit has been described with "coral calcium" that has a lower magnesium content (see: the product Halstead Coral Calcium™ and the book entitled *Fossil Stony Coral Minerals and Their Nutritional Application*, by B. W. Halstead MD, 1999) (available at www.wellnesspublishing.com).

- The nutritional benefits of coral calcium may, or may not, be enhanced by the addition of co-factors such as vitamins and other specific trace elements that have a clear biological role in supporting body structures and functions (see Barefoot Coral Calcium Plus™, www.naturesbenefit.com). Adding digestive enzymes or plant enzymes to coral calcium supplements and claiming that they enhance mineral absorption is a marketing gimmick. Excessive doses of fat-soluble vitamins (D, A and K) should be avoided, as should toxic elements, e.g. cesium. [Earlier uses of terms "Coral Calcium Formula" may refer to the addition of vitamins, etc., and the product Barefoot Coral Calcium Plus™ was formulated by a physician not by Mr. Robert Barefoot.]

- Coral calcium supplements must use material that is free from toxic metals and organic pollutants found in the ocean (e.g. lead, mercury, cadmium, PCBs, see www.naturesbenefit.com). Substances with unknown actions or lack of demonstrated synergy with coral calcium should not be added to supplements e.g. cesium and plant enzymes.

- Mr. Barefoot speaks about a formula but his additions to coral calcium supplements are arbitrary. There is no recorded proprietary coral calcium supplement formula. The concept of a "formula" is valueless; the most important factor is the use of high quality coral. Mr. Barefoot has not consistently endorsed one type of coral calcium or even one formula!

- Coral calcium supplements should contain coral calcium material for which there is a clear precedent of benefit. This benefit is described at least equally with land-based and below-sea level coral calcium (see the writings of Dr. Beth Ley, Mr. Barefoot or those of Dr. B Halstead MD at www.wellnesspublishing.com). Most scientific work has been performed on the below-sea level collected coral calcium, which is allegedly balanced with a ratio of calcium to magnesium of 2:1 (see Chapter 6).

- In terms of effectiveness, land-based and below-sea level coral appears to be equivalent in described benefits, but many of these benefits are anecdotal descriptions. Research is emerging with below-sea collected coral calcium (see Chapters 5 and 6).

- Only coral remnants that are collected with due attention to the support of the environment should be used in coral calcium supplements, regardless of whether or not they are collected from land or sea (www.naturesbenefit.com).

- There is no precedent for the use of soft gel capsules or tablets or caplets to deliver coral calcium. Tablets or caplets of coral calcium may not have the favorable absorption and dissolution characteristics of capsules and they must, at this stage, be avoided.

On the basis of the above statements, I propose what I believe to be optimum formulae for coral calcium supplements, which are sold by Natures Benefit Inc. (see www.naturesbenefit.com). The formulae that I propose differ from several common recommendations in the dietary supplement market, notably by my recommendation of at a least 1.5 g of whole coral calcium, underwater-based (Barefoot Coral Calcium Plus™ or Marine Coral Minerals™ www.naturesbenefit.com) or land-based coral calcium (Halstead Coral Calcium™ or Coral Calcium Powder™, www.naturesbenefit.com). One could argue that all additions to coral calcium are arbitrary and even that they are irrational. Certainly, the addition of significant amounts of cesium, an element that is potentially toxic and has no biological role, is quite reckless, let alone completely irrational. Three of the four formulations that I propose have no vitamin additions. **I stress that high-quality land- and below-sea collected coral are both potentially beneficial supplements, contrary to marketing propaganda.**

Some manufacturers avoid the use of adequate amounts of coral calcium in their supplements, because higher doses of coral calcium obviously increase the cost of the product, typically by at least 30%. This situation takes margins out of their sales. There are some companies that add calcium carbonate to coral calcium and label the product "coral calcium." I believe that this is materially misleading and false labeling. While the dietary supplement facts panel on some products that are "cut" with calcium carbonate shows higher calcium content, consumers should know that the calcium they are taking in these cheaper products is not originating in total from coral calcium. In some cases, I support a co-administration of vitamins E, D, A and C with coral calcium for their obvious health benefits; this type of combination is found in Barefoot Coral Calcium Plus™, but I stress the power of the product is in the quality of the coral, not in the arbitrary recommendations for vitamins and other additives (www.naturesbenefit.com). **The idea that there is a "supreme" or "superior" formula of coral calcium out there is nonsense.**

Vitamin D is essential for calcium absorption (in part) and utilization in the body, but high dosages <u>must</u> be avoided, contrary to some "popular", but misguided recommendations. Further, I recommend in some formulations the addition of certain micronutrient metals that have a well-defined role in health, notably selenium, zinc, boron, chromium and molybdenum. I do not support the use of significant amounts of metals or elements such as cesium, nickel or silver in coral calcium formulations, even though <u>small</u> doses may be harmless. How important it is to present the coral calcium in a balance of calcium to magnesium of two parts calcium to one part magnesium, remains debatable, but this form has received more recent research and development effort than other forms of coral calcium. Coral calcium balanced in a ratio of Ca:Mg of 2:1 is available in Barefoot Coral Calcium Plus™ and Marine Coral Minerals™ in doses of 1.5 grams per day.

Concerning the specific coral calcium content of supplements, I recommend the use of both land-collected and below-sea collected coral (of high quality) for many of the reasons defined earlier. Consumers must be given choices. My recommendations have been developed by a combination of feedback on reported individual benefits, often studied in an uncontrolled manner, and interpretation of what is known to be factual about coral calcium supplements. The formulae that I recommend are described in table 3 as Supplement Facts panels. In these coral calcium products, at least 1.5 g of high-quality coral calcium is recommended daily. These products deliver more 100% pure coral calcium than most other brands and they have experienced more continued use and re-order than any other brand of coral calcium in the U.S. market. In fact, millions of unit-dosages of coral calcium supplements made by Natures Benefit Inc. have been used with customer satisfaction and high re-order rate. The high re-order rate of dietary supplements is always a result of perceived benefits by consumers. Many coral calcium supplements have appeared in the market with labels that are only weeks old and they have no precedent of benefits.

BOTH LAND AND BELOW SEA LEVEL-COLLECTED CORAL CALCIUM ARE BENEFICIAL HOLISTIC MINERAL SUPPLEMENTS

Marine Coral Minerals™: Servings per container: 30, Serving Size: 3 capsules contain:

100% High Grade Coral Calcium from Okinawa, Japan	1500 mg
Calcium (26% RDI)	360 mg
Magnesium (45% RDI) from coral magnesium carbonate	180 mg

With trace minerals with natural variability including: selenium, zinc, copper, potassium, iodine, iron and up to 70 other mineral elements In parts per million Other ingredients: Silicon dioxide, cellulose, magnesium stearate and gelatin. No cholesterol, fat and calories.

Coral Calcium Powder™: Servings per container: 30, Serving Size: 3 g (one scoop) contains:

	Amount Per Serving	% Daily Value
High Grade Coral Calcium from Okinawa, Japan	3 g	N/A
Calcium (from coral)	1200 mg	120%
Magnesium (from coral)	30 mg	7.5%

Also contains many minerals or elements up to 70 or so with natural variability.

Halstead Stony Coral Minerals Coral Calcium™: Servings per container: 30, Serving Size: 3 capsules contain:

	Amount per Serving	% Daily Value
Stony Coral Minerals from Okinawa, Japan	1500 mg	N/A
Calcium from Coral Calcium	600 mg	60%
Magnesium from Coral Calcium	15 mg	3.5%

Also contain many minerals or elements up to 70 or so with natural variability.

Barefoot Coral Calcium Plus™: Servings per container: 30, Serving Size: 3 capsules contain:

	Amount Per Serving	% Daily Value
Coral Calcium (up to 70 trace minerals and elements with natural variability)	1500 mg	
Vitamin C (as Ascorbic Acid)	60 mg	100%
Vitamin D3 (as Cholecalciferol)	400 IU	100%
Vitamin E (natural)	30 IU	100%
Vitamin A	2197 IU	44%
Calcium (from coral calcium)	380 mg	36%
Iodine (Kelp)	10 mcg	7%
Magnesium	180 mg	45%
Zinc (as Zinc Oxide)	15 mg	100%
Selenium (as amino acid chelate)	20 mcg	29%
Copper (as amino acid chelate)	30 mcg	2%
Manganese (as amino acid chelate)	10 mcg	<1%
Chromium (as amino acid chelate)	120 mcg	100%
Molybdenum (as amino acid chelate)	10 mcg	13%
Vanadium (as amino acid chelate)	30 mcg	*
Boron (as amino acid chelate)	20 mcg	*

* Daily Value not established / 2:1 Calcium:Magnesium Ratio

Table 3: This table describes the Supplements Facts panels on some of the leading brands of coral calcium sold in the United States. Information was supplied with the permission of Natures Benefit Inc. www.naturesbenefit.com. Note Mr. Barefoot does not have a "proprietary formula" as such; his name was originally linked to high quality coral calcium products with or without arbitrary additions. Natures Benefit Inc. does not add cesium to its products.

CORAL CALCIUM WITH ADDED CESIUM IS BEST AVOIDED FOR POTENTIAL SAFETY PROBLEMS

READING LABELS

I have displayed the formulae contained in typical supplement facts panel in table 2, in order to help consumers understand how to interpret the average coral calcium dietary supplement label. Readers should please note that the amount of calcium listed on the supplement facts label (legal requirements) differs from the total amount of coral calcium in the product. This is simply because coral calcium is <u>much more than just calcium.</u> It is a mixture of coral debris (ash) containing other minerals and elements elaborated by the living coral or delivered from biogenous sediments on the ocean floor. Analyses of coral calcium show up to 74 different micromineral associated elements.

MORE ABOUT COMBINING NUTRIENTS WITH CORAL

The use of combined formulas of coral calcium with other vitamins and elements is very popular, but many people already take multivitamins or other supplements, such that they are better suited to taking coral calcium alone. For this circumstance, I recommend products that have no vitamin additives (e.g. Marine Coral Minerals™, Halstead Coral Calcium™ and Coral Calcium Powder™). These coral calcium products are present in capsules or a powder without vitamin additives. Coral Calcium Powder™ is pure coral powder, taken with a scoop and added to food or liquid, in a dose of up to 3 g/day. This form of coral calcium supplement is similar in its delivery with the traditional use of coral calcium food supplements in Japan.

I reiterate that excessive intake of vitamins D, A and K are to be avoided. Vitamin K has been added to some coral calcium supplements, but I consider this to be unnecessary because most requirements are met for vitamin K by its synthesis on the large bowel and its intake in the average diet. Furthermore, vitamin K affects blood clotting and excessive supplementation could increase risks of bleeding, especially in people receiving blood-thinning medications. Adding enzymes to coral calcium is of doubtful value. The co-administration of betaine with coral calcium is probably not advantageous.

CHAPTER SUMMARY

Consumers of coral calcium have been confused by marketing propaganda. A rational basis can be proposed for appropriate dosages and formats of coral calcium supplements, but many of these supplements have irrational formulations. The idea or concept of a "superior" formula of coral calcium, based on arbitrary additions of other "nutrients" is not valid. The primary issue is the type and amount of coral calcium used. Supplement products with a relatively long precedent of use are to be preferred (www.naturesbenefit.com). Excessive vitamin intake is to be avoided, especially vitamin D; and cesium taken in milligram amounts is potentially toxic in susceptible individuals. Powders and capsules of coral calcium must be preferred over soft gels or tablets (caplets) for which there is no clear precedent of benefit.

**AVOID CORAL CALCIUM PRODUCTS
WITH ADDED CESIUM**
www.coralcalciummagazine.com
www.gsdl.com

CHAPTER 4:

BIOLOGICAL AND BIOCHEMICAL FUNCTIONS OF CORAL CALCIUM

HOW DOES CORAL CALCIUM WORK? THE CORRECTION OF MINERAL DEPLETION?

Much speculation exists on how coral calcium may exert a health benefit. It is clear that many elements and minerals are necessary for the support of vital body structures and functions, and the mere act of supplementing minerals is often regarded as health-giving. Enzyme systems in the body, which help to control the chemistry of life often contain or require specific elements as co-factors, in order that they can operate efficiently. **A co-factor in the chemistry of life can be a metal or a vitamin.** For example, calcium exerts effects on many body functions including how muscles contract, how the heart beats and even how messages of life are transmitted to cells. These actions of calcium permit the body to function in a normal manner. The same is true of many other elements or minerals, e.g. magnesium, zinc, selenium, etc. (Table 4). The effects of elements on driving the chemistry of life are clear when one inspects the role of certain elements in the synthesis and breakdown of large molecules that are essential to life; and one discovers the essential role of elements in producing energy for life (Table 4).

THE ROLE OF CERTAIN
ELEMENTS IN BODY CHEMISTRY

BREAKDOWN OF MACROMOLECULES	SYNTHESIS OF MACROMOLECULES
Glucose entering Krebs cycle: Chromium, Cobalt, Copper, Magnesium, Manganese, Potassium, Zinc	Glycogen: Calcium, Chlorine, Magnesium, Potassium
Fatty acids entering Krebs cycle:	Fatty acids forming lipids:
Magnesium, Sulfur	Magnesium, Manganese
Amino acids entering Krebs cycle:	Amino acids forming proteins:
Magnesium, Potassium	Magnesium

KREBS CYCLE GENERATING ENERGY AND BYPRODUCTS

Requires calcium, cobalt, copper, iron, magnesium, manganese, potassium and zinc for function.

Table 4: This table is modified from data presented in Human Biology by DJ. Farish (Jones and Bartlett Publishers, Boston, 1993). Minerals (elements) are necessary co-factors for body chemistry and they are part of many enzymes involved in metabolism. This means that minerals are required for the assembly of large organic molecules in the body. In particular, minerals are needed to convert the molecules that enter the chains of chemical reactions in the body that produce energy (e.g. the Krebs cycle). Furthermore, certain elements have to be present for the function of the chemical cycles in the body that produce energy (the Krebs cycle). At the very least, adequate mineral intake must be considered "energizing". The most common report of benefit of coral calcium is that people "feel generally better" with "more energy". These anecdotal benefits seem to be consistent with the vital role of elements in the chemistry of life, but I stress that anecdotes are not scientific proof of effects.

Chemical analyses of several types of coral calcium show that it contains up to 74 different elements derived from the earth's crust and elaborated originally by live coral polyps from sea water. **The mineral content of the human body includes all minerals that occur in nature to variable degrees.** Calcium is a dominant element in the body of many living organisms, but it is not the only important nutrient mineral (Table 4). The importance of mineral supplementation has been magnified by reports that mineral deficiencies in Western society may be much more common than people realize. Evidence has emerged that our immediate environment may be considered to be "depleted" of minerals and certain key elements. "Clever" food processing has robbed minerals from the average Western diet.

Much agricultural land has been farmed extensively and a number of nutrient deficiencies in soils are described. Since plants derive their final composition from the soil, factors such as mineral deficiency may lead to a lower nutrient value of some fruits and vegetables. Further, several types of mineral or elemental deficiency are clearly associated with diseases in humans. For example, zinc deficiency has been associated with poor immune function. In addition, zinc is necessary for the function of the hormone insulin. Furthermore, insulin function is a major issue for public health, given the occurrence of the metabolic syndrome X, obesity, hypertension, high blood cholesterol and insulin resistance in up to 70 million American people (see Holt S, *Combat Syndrome X, Y and Z...*, www.wellnesspublishing.com). These are examples of the essential nature of certain micronutrient metals (Table 4).

There are many other examples of how elements, available as minerals, promote well-being, e.g. boron for bone health, magnesium for cardiovascular function, chromium for insulin function, etc. However, the amounts of many micronutrient metals found in coral calcium are quite small. **The small concentrations of many minerals in coral calcium do not defeat all arguments in favor of the potential effectiveness of coral calcium for health.** Indeed, the "cell salt theory" which is an extension of homeopathic medicine (see Schuessler's Theory, Chapter 5) provides support for the claims of health benefits of small concentrations of supplemented minerals. Schuessler's Theory is based on "biochemic" principals, but these theories have not been embraced by all physicians.

A REVIEW OF MINERALS AND HEALTH

Although 90 naturally occurring elements exist, the biological importance of only 25 or so is clearly recognized. However, modern research has suggested a potential biological role for small amounts of other elements (in excess of 25). One striking example of this situation is the role of minute amounts of arsenic (a poison) in the body. Strange as it may seem, minute doses of arsenic may have some beneficial roles in the chemistry of life. These new findings must not be interpreted as a reason to promote the use of potentially toxic elements in the diet, where the biological role of such elements is not clear, because serious toxicity and even death are dangers. These arguments must apply to the recent irrational use of milligram amounts of cesium in some coral calcium supplements.

I reiterate that recent trends in alternative medicine to use potentially toxic doses of "alkaline" elements such as cesium must be viewed with caution. Such recommendations have no role whatsoever in general health promotion, even though they may be of experimental interest (see chapter 7).

I have used the words element and mineral as interchangeable, but this is strictly not correct. Nutritionists have tended to refer to the actions of elements by calling them minerals. However, an element in one specific chemical form can be beneficial, whereas the same element in a different chemical form can be toxic (e.g. chromium). **The four most important elements of life are hydrogen, nitrogen, carbon and oxygen;** the other 21 are categorized as either macronutrient minerals or micronutrient minerals (Tables 5 and 6).

MACROELEMENT	FUNCTION
SODIUM	Water balance, glucose handling and nervous system functions.
POTASSIUM	Water balance, protein synthesis, nerve cell functions, cardiac and smooth muscle function.
CHLORINE	Regulator of acid-base balance, tissue growth, digestive function (gastric acid) and intestinal secretions.
CALCIUM	Blood clotting, bone and teeth structure and function, activity of many metabolic enzymes, muscle structure and function, protein synthesis.
PHOSPHORUS	Energy production, bones and teeth function of cell membranes, functions of genetic material (nucleic acid structure) and glucose handling.
MAGNESIUM	Important co-factor for metabolic enzymes, bones and teeth, smooth muscle activity, cardiac muscle function.

Table 5: A summary of the main function of the seven macroelements that are obligatory in the diet for health maintenance.

There is a vast amount of literature on the biological effects of nutrient minerals and their presence in the human diet is as essential to life as any vitamin. There is no doubt that medicine has focused much attention on vitamin intake at the expense of considering the essential (obligatory) nature of macroelements and microelements (the minerals). The roles of macroelements, (found in relatively large amounts in the body), and the roles of microelements (found in tiny amounts), are summarized in Tables 5 and 6. This brief review of mineral nutrients is important in our understanding of how holistic natural minerals supplements, such as coral calcium, may exert potent and versatile health benefits.

MICROELEMENT FUNCTION

IRON	Supports electron transport systems, mitochondrial function, enzyme co-factor and critical component of hemoglobin.
ZINC	Hormone function (insulin), wound healing, digestive enzyme functions, bone, immune function.
FLUORINE	Calcium metabolism, bones and teeth (arguable benefits).
IODINE	Thyroid gland function and component of thyroid hormone.
SELENIUM	An antioxidant metal, cardiac muscle function, teeth, supports actions of vitamin E.
MANGANESE	Connective tissue function, bone function, supports several metabolic enzymes.
COPPER	Nervous system, liver function, blood, connective tissue and enzyme co-factor.
MOLYBDENUM	Enzyme co-factor, essential.
CHROMIUM	Insulin function, glucose metabolism.
COBALT	A component of vitamin B12 with many actions, e.g. blood and CNS.
NICKEL	Nucleic acid metabolism and correct handling of iron in the body.
VANADIUM	Fat and iron metabolism, bone development, function of insulin and growth of tissues.

SILICON   Connective tissue growth, development and integrity.

TIN   Involved in tissue growth.

Table 6: A summary of microminerals (or microelements) that are essential for many body structures and functions. In general, these elements are needed in much smaller quantities than the macronutrient minerals (or elements) listed in Table 5. Note that cesium is not a "nutrient" element.

MINERAL REQUIREMENTS ARE DEBATED

The optimal amount of intake of various minerals in a healthy diet has been subject to much debate. Many contemporary nutritionists feel that recommended daily intake (RDI) of certain vitamins or minerals is insufficient for many people. Authors of popular books on the subject of vitamin and mineral supplements stress that recommended daily allowances (or recommended daily intakes, RDI) of vital nutrients are designed only to prevent deficiencies of nutrients. Conventional recommendations for "healthy" mineral intake have been subject to continuing revision. Certainly, recommended daily intakes of calcium for health have been increased over the past few years (Table 7) and modern research points to a biological action of several microelements (Table 6) that were formerly thought to be non-essential.

Stage of Life (in mg of calcium)	Optimal Daily Intake
WOMEN	
25-50 years	1000
Pregnant and nursing	1200-1500
Over 50 years post-menopausal	
On estrogens	1000
Not on estrogens	1500
Over 65 years	1500
MEN	
25-65 years	1000
Over 65 years	1500

ADOLESCENTS/YOUNG ADULTS
11-24 years   1200-1500

CHILDREN
Up to 10 years   800-1200

INFANTS
Up to 1 year   400-600

Table 7: Optimal calcium requirements during an individual's lifetime. These data are taken from NIH Consensus Statement, Vol. 12, No. 4, June 6-8, 1994. Note: These estimates have been raised upward in some circumstances and I believe that there is evidence to even further increase recommended intakes of calcium.

Shari Lieberman PhD and Nancy Bruning (authors of *The Real Vitamin & Mineral Book*) have proposed that not all nutrients can be obtained from today's regular food supplies. These authors stress that recommended daily intakes (RDI) of minerals vary considerably among individuals and that current recommended mineral intake may not guarantee optimal health. Further, these authors imply that extensive food tables describing the nutrient value of certain foods tend to overestimate nutrient contents of many foods. The analogy used by Dr. Lieberman and Ms. Bruning is that "like clothes," standard recommendations for mineral intake do not conform to the idea that "one size fits all." In other words, the concept of the RDI is not portable among the population. **There are different mineral needs for different people.** Despite the arguments, it is clear in scientific literature that certain vitamins and minerals afford protection against the development of disease; and in some cases they many even counteract the effect of some environmental pollution on health.

MINERALS: MORE OR LESS?

Many nutritionists claim that there is widespread micronutrient deficiency in the population, especially specific types of trace elements or minerals. However, one must not be too quick to assume that more is necessarily better, especially when it comes to vitamins and minerals. There are many experiments that show that excess amounts of certain minerals do not have a better effect on health than smaller amounts of intake (and vice versa). Moreover, some essential micronutrients and elements are toxic when given in excess. Thus, the proponents of excessive mineral intake for health have to be questioned. For example, selenium, which is recommended for its indirect antioxidant effects, and other benefits on health, can cause cardiovascular problems when taken in very high doses. In contrast, selenium in modest amounts can benefit cardiovascular health. It seems more than a coincidence that nature provides holistic mineral sources such as coral calcium with a comprehensive, but modest amount of many microelements.

In general, high doses of water-soluble vitamins, such as vitamin C (up to 5g/day, an amount much greater than RDI) are believed by many physicians to be relatively harmless. However, very high concentrations of vitamin C (greater than 5 grams per day) when given alone may have a negative health effect, by promoting, rather than preventing, oxidative stress in the body. The toxicity of fat-soluble vitamins in high dosages is not in question. More than the recommended daily intake of vitamin D, in the absence of vitamin D deficiency, cannot be considered health giving. In this regard, I disagree with recommendations for liberal vitamin D intake, unless it is supervised by a knowledgeable healthcare giver. In addition, excessive intake of vitamins A and K can have quite serious consequences. The consensus opinion in medicine is that large doses of fat-soluble vitamins (A, D, E and K) are to be avoided, except under special medical circumstances, where close supervision must occur.

I cannot question the proposal that mineral intake from coral calcium would be beneficial for many people who may be missing certain important macro- and microelements in their diets (Tables 5 and 6). Certainly, the micronutrient content of commonly eaten, processed food is constantly in question. Further, agricultural practices that are used to increase crop yields have been blamed as an indirect cause of nutrient deficiency in the population. A large proportion of the population has turned to mineral-depleted, fast food or junk food as a staple component of their diet. These circumstances may help foster widespread micronutrient (mineral) deficiency in modern society.

MINERAL SALTS AND HEALTH: POTENTIAL HOMEO-PATHIC EFFECTS OF CORAL CALCIUM

Coral calcium (marine or stony coral minerals etc.) appear to be an attractive holistic mineral supplement to many people, but this supplement may not necessarily exert its actions by the direct supply of commonly recommended amounts of certain nutrients (especially RDI). This reasoning applies to situations where desired amounts of minerals are defined as widely accepted, recommended daily intakes (RDI). I have suggested previously that coral calcium may work by a homeopathic mechanism. **This proposal may explain why people (e.g. Okinawans) taking coral calcium supplements that contain trace amounts of many elements or even drinking coral water, which contains very tiny amounts of many minerals, could have the benefits that have been described in some testimonials. Coral calcium minerals are relatively insoluble and they only dissolve in very small amounts in water. Coral calcium, in turn, contains only very small amounts of many minerals. This leads to the question: "Is coral water or coral calcium powder a homeopathic remedy?"**

Homeopathy is a medical specialty where very small doses of natural agents are used to treat a variety of diseases. A basic principle of homeopathic medicine is the use of "like to treat like" and inorganic materials (elements and minerals) are used in various types of homeopathy. One common form of homeopathy is called "lithotherapy", where dilutions of natural minerals or rocks (e.g., coral sand or coral) are used in treatment. One may ask further, "Is drinking coral water a form of homeopathic lithotherapy?"

I stress that very tiny amounts of minerals are present in homeopathic treatments. Lithotherapy is an extension of homeopathic treatments that have been used in Germany and other Western countries for many years. This type of therapy has been expanded by some researchers and referred to as "cell salt therapy," as originally proposed by W. Schuessler MD. Dr. Schuessler was a German physician who developed the "biochemic extensions" of homeopathic medicine. There have been modern accounts of the success of cell salt therapy and some extensions of this therapy have included the administration of a variety of minerals or elements in trace amounts. As we start to examine the specific chemical composition of coral calcium, the potential value of its contents of many elements in parts per million (very small amounts) will become apparent.

ORIGINS OF THE SUGGESTIONS OF THE IMPORTANCE OF BACTERIA IN CORAL CALCIUM

Before we delve further into the hypotheses of how coral calcium could exert a health benefit, certain fantasies must be further dispelled. As previously discussed, some professed experts on coral calcium claim that microorganisms (said to be present in coral calcium) play a role in the beneficial effects of coral calcium supplements for health. Reflect upon the descriptions of the processing of coral, which is designed to render coral sand as sterile as possible. One may see immediately the absurdity of this suggestion concerning the presence or actions of "microbes" in coral supplements. It has been stated that microorganisms in coral may help gastrointestinal function and "hearsay" suggests that this theory was proposed by Scandinavian scientists. I can find no evidence to support this preposterous suggestion. Coral calcium is free of bacteria. However, E. Enby MD, a Scandinavian physician, has proposed that much chronic disease may be related to undiscovered infections in the body and he has linked this hypothesis to the presence of chronic acidity in the body. I believe that the confusion concerning the role of microorganisms, linked to coral calcium, may be an ignorant interpretation of Dr. Enby's assertions and work. However, Dr. Enby has opinions that may not be shared by all practicing physicians.

BODY ACIDITY AND ALKALINITY

The whole issue of body acidity and alkalinity has become an issue of great debate in alternative and conventional medicine. Many practitioners of alternative medicine believe that modern lifestyle is pushing many people to a body status of acidity (low pH). Modern proponents of high body pH (alkali) therapy argue that controlling body pH in the upper range is healthy-giving. In contrast, one may reflect on folklore medicine that has proposed the benefits of acid therapies, such as apple cider vinegar (See Marsh EE, "How to be Healthy with Natural Foods", Gramercy Publishers, NY, MCMLXIII). It has been proposed that mineral intake, especially intake of "alkaline" metals (e.g. calcium), may assist in neutralizing the body acidity in a beneficial manner. **It has even been suggested that mineral intake may cause the body to become more alkaline.** These hypotheses are very interesting, but they are not universally accepted as clinically significant in modern medicine. I question their significance.

The body has very complex mechanisms that control acidity and alkalinity (pH balance in the body). Certainly this balance has much to do with many factors, other than mineral intake in the diet. With some naivete, people have recommended the simplistic monitoring of the pH of certain body fluids (saliva and urine). Further, some individuals have proposed that not only can body pH be influenced by mineral intake, one can give desirable amounts of minerals by gauging their effect on the pH of body fluids. I believe that this notion of mineral supplementation by crude tests of body pH is far-fetched and it only serves the sale pH-monitoring gadgets of limited value (pH testing kits) a waste of time and money?

It must be recognized that body fluids have changes in pH (a measure of the presence of hydrogen ions, or acid) on a regular basis. For example, urine becomes alkaline after a meal. This is known in basic physiology as the "alkaline tide." Therefore, selling strips of paper (litmus paper) or gadgets to measure pH of body fluids, as a way of monitoring the intake of minerals supplements has to be questioned. I am not suggesting that some minerals may not have a modest and positive influence on increasing body pH, but I am suggesting that the influence is small in comparison to the many other systems in the body that act as the primary buffers of acid (promoting alkalinity or rise in the pH of some body fluids). Furthermore, I believe that selling products on the basis of balancing pH by using gadgets to measure body pH, such as litmus paper strips, is quite misleading. Several scientists reject the Acid/Alkaline Theory of Disease as nonsense. In my mind, the "jury remains out" on this type of therapy. In fact, the only body fluid pH that appears to be affected materially by diet or dietary supplements is the urine.

The main theories of how coral calcium works can be summarized as follows; a general natural holistic mineral supplement, or a homeopathic agent, or cell salt therapy, or as a regulator of body pH. I would add to these proposals the fact there may be other actions of coral calcium that remain undiscovered. Of the proposed mechanisms of action for coral calcium and health, I favor the explanation of the value of coral calcium as a natural mineral supplement. As a mineral supplement, I believe that it provides a wide range of available micronutrients (metals and minerals) that support many body structures and functions. This explanation makes the most sense as people increasingly report that they "just feel better" (a global anecdote) when they take coral calcium. However, my observations in this regard are based on anecdotes not controlled scientific studies.

The nonspecific reports of improvement and well-being after taking the dietary supplement coral calcium could be explained by the overall value of minerals for health, especially in individuals who may be depleted of several micronutrient elements. The rapid swing of pH demonstrated by adding coral calcium enclosed in a teabag to water may often be related to the addition of baking soda (sodium bicarbonate) to the coral calcium – a slick, sales trick! However, exposing coral calcium to water does produce alkaline, ionized water that may have health benefits (see Chapter 6).

HOW THE BODY CONTROLS ACIDITY AND ALKALINITY

The subject of pH balance is highly complex and I am attempting to simplify the issues for readers who do not have training in biomedical science. The control of body pH (acidity or alkalinity) is not easily understood by the layperson and sometimes by "healers". In recent times, practitioners of alternative medicine have reactivated early hypotheses on body acidity that were proposed in the late 19th and early 20th centuries. These hypotheses relate to chronic acidity of the body as a cause of degenerative diseases and cancer. Such hypotheses do have interesting but unproven potential in the explanation of the multiple causes of chronic disease. Furthermore, these hypotheses are dramatically opposite to some types of folklore (alternative) medicine.

The balance of acids and alkalis (bases) in the body centers around the precise control of hydrogen ions (H+) that float free in body water of the cells and body fluids: Acids are hydrogen (H+) containing substances which liberate free H+ groups that cause acidity. Strong acids give up hydrogen ions freely and weak acids are less potent in their donation of H+ (acid). In contrast, a base is a substance that can neutralize an acid. There are weak bases and strong bases that vary in their ability to bind hydrogen ions.

There is a very narrow range of acid or alkalinity with which life is compatible. The degree of acidity or alkalinity of body fluids is measured in pH. The pH value is related to the presence of H+ ions where high levels of H+ ions cause a low pH (acidity) and low levels of H+ ions cause a high pH (alkalinity). Thus, there is a reciprocal relationship between H+ concentrations and measures of pH. In fact, the relationship between H+ ions and pH is logarithmic.

Pure water has a pH of 7.0, but the pH of arterial blood is 7.45 and the pH of venous blood is more acid at pH 7.35. Death occurs rapidly if pH changes move out of the ranges of 6.8 to 8.0, a range from severe acidosis to severe alkalosis. Small changes in pH have a major effect on body chemistry and the healthy body has chemical mechanisms that maintain tight control over body pH. These are reasons to avoid self medication with highly alkaline elements such as cesium. Cesium is the most alkaline, electropositive element with no defined biological role in the human body. Table 8 summarizes some effects of altered body pH on the chemistry of life.

ACIDOSIS (Low pH)	ALKALOSIS (High pH)
Depression of CNS function	Over-excitability of the nervous system, cramps, pins and needles, muscle spasms and even convulsions.
Altered chemical shape and activity of the structure and function of metabolic enzymes	Altered chemical shape and activity of the structure and function of metabolic enzymes.
Altered concentrations of other minerals in the body e.g. high blood potassium	Altered concentrations of other minerals, e.g. low blood potassium

Table 8: The chemistry of life is affected to a major degree by shifts in pH (acidosis or alkalosis). Enzymes may act slower or faster, tissue oxygenation may change and shift in elements like potassium can cause cardiac problems. Some alternative medicine theory talks about minor changes in body acidity as a cause of chronic disease.

THE BODY PRODUCES ACID

Hydrogen ions are produced continuously by the body as a result of carbonic acid formation which is produced in turn from carbon dioxide combining with water. Acids are also produced by the breakdown of nutrients, especially protein-containing amino acids. When sulfur- and phosphorus-containing proteins are broken down sulfuric acid or phosphoric acid are produced. Thus, body acids result from normal metabolism. An example is the production of lactic acid from muscles during periods of significant exercise (a state of "minor" lactic acidosis).

The body has first, second and third lines of defenses to control body pH. These include buffer systems and the respiratory system and the kidneys. Changes in acid base balance (pH) in the body arise from changes in respiratory function or from metabolic disturbances. Thus, there can be respiratory acidosis, low pH in the blood, (e.g. chronic obstructive lung disease), respiratory alkalosis, high pH in the blood, (hyperventilation), metabolic acidosis (diarrhea, diabetes mellitus, strenuous exercise, kidney disease) and metabolic alkalosis (vomiting or taking excessive amounts of alkaline materials such as sodium bicarbonate or calcium carbonate). It can be understood how calcium carbonate intake can contribute to raising pH in body fluids because it tends to cause a metabolic type of alkalosis (high body pH), in simple terms.

A very high dose of calcium carbonate, sometimes with added milk, has resulted in a condition called the "milk alkali syndrome" (of Burnett). This is a serious disorder of body metabolism where kidney stones can occur. It is rarely encountered these days, but it was seen with outdated treatments for peptic ulcers, where very large amounts of calcium carbonate and milk were administered—an outdated treatment for peptic ulcer.

FIRST LINES OF BODY pH CONTROL

The body has a series of buffer systems that keep the constant production of H+ (acid) in check. These buffer systems "mop-up" acid. The most important buffers involve the carbonic acid/bicarbonate buffer system, the protein buffer system (involving cellular proteins and proteins in the blood), the hemoglobin buffer system and the phosphate buffer system. The chemical buffer systems in the body are constantly at work. The balance of body pH depends in part on the carbonic acid/bicarbonate buffer system in which the major mineral in coral calcium (calcium carbonate) can variably participate. The simplified chemical reactions that I describe explain why calcium carbonate from coral calcium (like sodium bicarbonate, in baking soda) can tend to cause alkalinity of body pH, but readers must appreciate that this is only a <u>small facet</u> of the body's complex mechanisms of acid/base balance.

CESIUM ADDITION TO CORAL CALCIUM IS DANGEROUS

Several physicians, nutritionists and consumers have become convinced about the benefits of raising body pH, especially to treat or prevent cancer. I stress that people who use potent remedies to engage "high body pH therapy", (especially significant amounts of cesium), may be "playing with fire". Coral calcium products containing significant amounts of added cesium are very "ill-founded" and may be toxic. Scientific studies show that cesium has no biological role and in significant quantities it is toxic (references: www.webelements.com,
www.worldbook.aol.com,
www.cdc.gov/niosh/rtecs/fk958940.html,
www.atsdr.cdc.gov/tfacts157.html
Refer to the information center of ATSDR, Agency for Toxic Substances and Disease Registry, call 1-888-422-8737, www.gsdl.com/news/connections/vol13/conn20010711.html, a report of serious cardiac toxicity, www.cesium-chloride.com.
Cesium may cause abnormalities in the blood, serious heart problems and death in high doses. Scientists at the University of Sheffield, UK, report that "Rats fed cesium in place of potassium in their diet die" (www.webelements.com). Dr. Walid I. Saliba, M.D. et al at

the Cleveland Clinical Foundation, advise physicians to be aware of the potentially "life-threatening" toxicity of cesium chloride, particularly in individuals vulnerable to heart palpitations and arrhythmias.

CESIUM CAUSES SERIOUS HEART PROBLEMS IN SUSCEPTIBLE INDIVIDUALS

Eminent researchers at the Cleveland Clinical Foundation reported the case of a 47 year old woman who suddenly collapsed at home and was taken to hospital as a medical emergency. EKG tests showed that this lady had life threatening abnormalities of heart rhythm which was believed to be due to the taking of cesium chloride in the presence of low blood potassium. This report of serious toxicity due to cesium contained in a dietary supplement was reported in prestigious medical literature, (reference Saliba W, Erdogan O, Niebauer M. Polymorphic Ventricular Tachycardia in a Woman Taking Cesium Chloride. Pacing Clin Electrophysiol 2001; 24[pt I]:515-517).

AVOIDING CESIUM

Several responsible retailers and distributors of supplements have rejected coral calcium products with significant amounts of added cesium. While small amounts of cesium may be relatively safe, other coral calcium products with mg amounts of cesium must be considered very risky for general use by the public.

I can see no reason whatsoever to take the risk of adding milligram amounts of cesium to coral calcium given the evidence of its toxicity. In fact, the National Institute for Occupational Safety and Health (NIOSH) recommends a limit of 2 milligrams of cesium hydroxide per cubic meter of air (2mg /m3) as an average for a 10-hour work day, 40-hour work week.

CESIUM : A DOUBTFUL CANCER TREATMENT

Cesium belongs to a specific group of elements in the periodic table that possess similar properties. This group includes cesium, sodium, lithium and potassium and they have been referred to as "alkaline elements" by some nutritionists, perhaps with some degree of naivety. It is clear that the administration of cesium, lithium and potassium in significant amounts can alter the chemical environment of the body in a critical manner, especially the "ionic" status of cells.

About eighty years ago cesium and other elements were proposed as potential cancer treatments, but scientific studies as early as the 1930's failed to show any significant anticancer effects of cesium (Burton TS, Marsh MC, Annals of Surgery, 93, 169-179, 1931). However, it was discovered in the 1970's that certain cancer cells had an affinity for cesium and interest in cesium as a tumor therapy was reactivated. It was Dr. A.K. Brewer MD who proposed a technique for cancer treatment termed "high pH therapy" in the 1980's. Dr. Brewer administered very high doses of cesium chloride to mice and humans (6 grams per day to cancer patients) and reported some favorable, but inconsistent outcomes (Brewer AK, Phar.Biochem and Behavior, 21, 1, 1-5, 1984). However, in lower dosages of cesium (less than 3gm/day), Dr. Brewer noted actual increases in tumor growth. This experiment suggests that in some circumstances mildly elevating cell pH may promote cancer! Thus, giving smaller, but still potentially toxic doses of cesium may be the wrong thing to do? Clearly, without further clear guidelines the use of milligram amounts of cesium in dietary supplements is best avoided.

How cesium works in the body to produce any effect, toxic or otherwise, is not completely clear. Cesium can variably substitute itself for potassium in body chemistry and interfering with the function of potassium in the body is very critical to many key organ functions, especially cardiac function. John Boik in his excellent book on "Cancer and Natural Medicine" (Oregon Medical Press, 1995) suggests that optimizing the balance between cesium chloride and potassium is critical to the anticancer effect of cesium. I add that this balance is also a key to the toxicity of cesium; and individuals with altered blood potassium status (hypokalemia) may be very susceptible to the toxicity of cesium.

In one study, Dr. Sartori administered very high dosages of cesium chloride (6-9 grams per day) to patients with advanced cancer. These patients also received other alternative therapy with DMSO, minerals and vitamins. The results were inconclusive

(Sartori HE, Phar. Biochem and Behavior, 21, 1, 11-13, 1984). While about 50% of the patients survived a year (an inconclusive result), one half of the patients who died did so in the first two weeks of the study. This may mean that the cesium treatment could have caused their death (Boik J, Cancer and Natural Medicine, Oregon Press 1995).

Side effects of cesium administration include nausea, diarrhea and general gastrointestinal distress. It can cause both excitement and depression of the function of the central nervous system. In addition, it can stimulate cholinergic nerves and cause a rise in blood pressure, excess salivation, urination and piloerection (hair standing on end). Furthermore, cesium could, over time, accumulate in the body and substitute itself for potassium leading to potassium deficiency and heart toxicity. Clearly, significant quantities of cesium in dietary supplements have no role and they carry potential risks (see Pinsky C, Bose R, Phar.Biochem and Behavior, 21, 1, 17-23, 1984).

HIGH pH THERAPIES : THE OTHER SIDE OF THE COIN?

It may come as a shock to some of the believers in "high pH therapy" (body alkalinization) that anticancer effects of "low pH therapy" are well described in medical literature. It is known that low tissue oxygen concentrations and high cellular pH (alkalinity) potentially increase lactic acidosis; and, by inference, low cellular pH (acidity) or increase in oxygenation may inhibit cancer growth. Mr. Barefoot has suggested that alkalinity and calcium increase tissue oxygenation—both absurd comments not rooted in science. Calcium has no role in oxygen delivery and body acidity (especially low blood pH) favors oxygen donation to tissues. In brief, the occurrence of body acidity (systemic acidosis) has been suggested as a status that may promote cancer regression (Boik J, Cancer and Natural Medicine, Oregon Press, 1995 and Harguindey S, Medical Pediatric Oncology, 10, 217-36, 1982).

It is clear in scientific literature that the manipulation of body pH is a complex, "double -edged sword" and without meticulous medical supervision, it should not be used. Certainly, it is not a viable option for self-treatment. I am not convinced that coral calcium works to a major degree by altering body pH and I trust that many people will research this subject more and come to similar conclusions.

ANALYZING CORAL CALCIUM

Preceding authoritative, but somewhat outdated accounts of the analysis of fossilized, stony coral minerals, are to be found in the book entitled *Fossil Stony Coral Minerals and Their Nutritional Application* by Bruce Halstead MD (available at www.wellnesspublishing.com). The analyses of coral calcium performed by Dr. Halstead show most elemental contents in parts per million, except for calcium and magnesium. Dr. Halstead has summarized a comparison of major elements found in the Earth's crust, seawater, human body and stony coral fossils and he has reviewed the essential biological roles of the many trace elements found in coral minerals (www.halsteadcoralcalcium.com). In brief, Dr Halstead believed that many elements in coral calcium could support body structures and functions.

THE MICRONUTRIENT CONTENT OF CORAL CALCIUM

While much has been made out of the importance of the calcium and magnesium content of coral calcium, much less discussion has focused on the micronutrient mineral content of coral calcium. Both marine coral calcium and land-based coral calcium have a wide range of elements (up to 70, approx.). In fact, land-based coral has been shown to have up to 74 different elements on careful chemical analysis and below sea-collected coral sand may contain a similar range of elements (www.naturesbenefit.com, www.coralcalciuminformation.com, www.halsteadcoralcalcium.com, www.coralcalciummagazine.com).

Some researchers argue strongly that the micronutrient profile of land-based coral may be superior to marine coral, or vice versa. This is an unresolved debate. For example, it has been suggested by some that land-based coral is inferior in mineral content, due to weathering and drying that causes leaching of metals and minerals. Examples of global micronutrient analysis showing the content of various elements in coral is shown in Table 9. These data are recent (September 2001 and 2002) and they supersede other published material. Furthermore, I believe the results to be particularly valuable because they were done by independent laboratories with no commercial interests in coral calcium.

BELOW-SEA COLLECTED CORAL (HIGH GRADE)

Calcium	20% or more
Magnesium	10% or more
Arsenic (as As)	2 ppm or less
Heavy metal (as Ph)	0.5 ppm or less
Size of Particle	90% at 40 microns or less
Pesticide residue	Undetectable (Endrin, Dildrin, Aldorin, BHC, DDT)
<Microorganisms>	
General bacteria count	3 x 10 (3)/g or less
Yeast	1 x 10 (2)/g or less
Mold	1 x 10 (2)/g or less
Colibacillus	Negative
Salmonella	Negative
Vibrio (enteric)	Negative

ABOVE SEA LEVEL-COLLECTED CORAL CALCIUM (HIGH GRADE)

Calcium	35% or greater
Magnesium	6000 ppm or greater
Total minerals and elements	74 or greater
Lead	0.5 ppm or less
Mercury	0.1 ppm or less
Cadmium	0.3 ppm or less
Arsenic	0.5 ppm or less
Pesticide residue	Undetectable
Salmonella	Negative
Yeast	<10 cfu/g
Mold	<10 cfu/g
Total Coliform	<10 cfu/g
E. coli	<10 cfu/g

Table 9: The mineral profile and other relevant analyses of the content of the two highest grades of coral calcium used in dietary supplements. The data was supplied with the permission of Natures Benefit Inc. (www.naturesbenefit.com). Both below-sea collected coral calcium and coral calcium collected above ground contain up to 70 or more micronutrient elements or minerals with natural marine variability. This micronutrient profile of types of coral calcium is displayed on the web page (www.naturesbenefit.com). Many elements found in the earth's crust are present in all forms of coral remnants and they are most frequently present in very small amounts, measured in parts per million. The forms of land-collected coral remnants used by Natures Benefit Inc. are obtained from Okinawa and ground and processed in the USA or Japan. This form of coral

is sterilized by ozone treatment or heat. Below sea coral sand is sterilized typically by heat.

CONCERNS ABOUT SPECIFICATIONS ON CORAL

While several sections of this short book may appear technical in its content, the information can be summarized in a simple manner. First, the apparent advantage of some types of below-sea collected coral appears to be a higher magnesium concentration. Second, there is an unresolved argument whether or not naturally balanced (Ca:Mg, 2:1) coral sand exists. Third, the situation of low magnesium concentrations in some forms of coral calcium can be remedied often by adding magnesium to coral if required. Fourth, the reported health benefits from both types of high-grade coral discussed in this book appear to be similar, but the below-sea collected coral calcium with an alleged natural Ca:Mg of 2:1 has undergone more contemporary in vitro and in vivo research than land-based coral. Fifth, concerns must remain if manufacturers use below-sea collected coral with excessive lead or other heavy metals. Sixth, adding milligram amounts of cesium to coral calcium in supplements is not justified and it adulterates coral calcium.

MOVING TOWARDS THE IDEAL CORAL CALCIUM SUPPLE-MENTS

How does this information translate to a recommendation for an ideal coral calcium supplement? The answer rests in considering the relative advantages or limitations of different types of coral calcium. Therefore, it seems most appropriate for healthcare consumers to be offered land-based coral of high quality (e.g. Halstead Coral Calcium™ or Coral Calcium Powder™) and below-sea coral of high quality to provide the consumer with choices and the relative advantages of both types of coral calcium (Barefoot Coral Calcium Plus™ or Marine Coral Minerals™). Accepting that not all advantages and disadvantages of either type of coral calcium may have been recognized to date (see www.naturesbenefit.com). Unfortunately, the many emerging types of coral calcium supplements do not contain "tried and trusted" types of coral calcium of high grade (www.naturesbenefit.com) and some are labeled in a misleading manner. More than one hundred brands of coral calcium were present in the market at the time of writing and many of these appeared in a six month period starting September 2002. The precedent was set with capsules and powders not with tablets, caplets or soft gels. Consumers are advised to select a coral calcium supplement that has been in the market for a while where some history of safety and satisfaction exists. The idea or notion of a specific "formula" is not the issue; it is the quality of the coral calcium in the supplement that is important.

CORAL CALCIUM-CONTAINING TEABAGS

There has been a limited tradition in Western society of taking coral in novel or unusual formats. One popular way of taking coral is to drink coral water that has been exposed to a teabag containing coral calcium powder with additives (sometimes simple sodium bicarbonate, or baking soda). The addition of silver to tea bag enclosed coral is of no value or consequence. Some promoters of coral calcium have been very critical of this use of coral calcium in teabags even though they may have once supported this form of coral supplement (see the book *"Barefoot on Coral Calcium: An Elixir of Life"*, www.wellnesspublishing.com). At first sight, criticism of the use of coral water compared with encapsulated coral calcium seems plausible, because only a small percentage of coral minerals from the teabag-enclosed coral calcium dissolves in the water (less than 2 % of minerals dissolved over a matter of hours). It is obvious that swallowing coral calcium in whole capsules or powders as food additives provides greater amounts of mineral nutrients for the body. However, the advantages of coral calcium-containing teabags must not be dismissed lightly.

Dr. Halstead has described the potential link between the presence of coral-enriched water in Okinawa and the longevity of the local population and so have other authors. It would appear that the water supply in several areas of Okinawa is exposed to coral sand or fossilized remnants as a natural filtering mechanism. Referring to the homeopathic theory of the action of coral calcium, it could be hypothesized that coral water, derived from coral-enclosed teabags, is a homeopathic medicine.

Many reported testimonials of the health benefits of using

water exposed to coral calcium-containing teabags have been displayed on the Internet. It is not clear, whether testimonials of the benefit of coral calcium in solid dosage forms (pills and powders) are confused with testimonials of health benefits from people using water treated with teabag-enclosed coral. I think that coral water is perceived by many people to be a convenient way of using coral calcium and coral calcium itself will assist in the removal of chlorine from water and tend to make the water alkaline. That said, emerging science supports the potential value of Coral Calcium Water™, a form of Alkaline Ionized Water™ (Coralyte™) (www.naturesbenefit.com).

DISSOLVING CORAL? WHAT NEXT?

Innovative manufacturers in Japan have now developed what they describe as a "dissolving-type" of coral calcium. This type of "dissolving coral" is sold in aluminum packages that are referred to as "coral calcium sticks." Apparently, this form of coral calcium has become popular in some European countries. I am puzzled by this product and even more puzzled by consumers, purveyors and self-proclaimed experts who think that coral calcium should dissolve completely in water. In collaboration with manufacturers, Natures Benefit, Inc. has produced a very "fine" form of coral calcium with a tiny particle size (micronized). This powderized fine coral calcium can be used to make Coral Calcium Water™ (Coralyte™).

Many minerals in coral calcium, e.g. calcium and magnesium, are in the carbonate form. Carbonated minerals are relatively insoluble. In more simple terms, one can understand that if stony coral was able to dissolve completely in water, then there would be no coral reefs in the ocean! Recently, tablets or caplets and special encapsulation processes (soft gels) have been used to make forms of coral calcium. I can see no advantage to coral calcium in soft gels, which have no history of use and no credible precedent of health benefits. Tablets or caplets of coral calcium may impede the absorption of coral calcium minerals.

CHAPTER SUMMARY

Coral calcium exerts putative biological functions as a dietary supplement as a consequence of its overall mineral content. Many mechanisms of action may operate with a holistic mineral supplement like coral calcium. Minerals are known to be important in the chemistry of life and deficiency states of nutritive minerals cause disease. Evidence exists that the human food chain may be depleted in minerals, especially in western countries. Whilst adequate diet calcium intake is an important public health target, the notion of a "Calcium Factor" is an inadequate way of viewing the benefits of coral calcium. Arbitrary "formulae" for coral calcium supplements are less important than the quality of coral calcium in the supplement and formulae containing added cesium in significant (mg) amounts are to be avoided because of potential and unknown toxicity.

CHAPTER 5:

POTENTIAL HEALTH BENEFITS OF CORAL CALCIUM

SOME KEY BIOLOGICAL ACTIONS OF CORAL COMPONENTS

Dr. Halstead has expressed the opinion that certain elements in coral minerals, such as deuterium and germanium, may have novel health benefits. Dr. Halstead describes the presence of an approximate level of deuterium of 150 parts per million in stony fossilized corals (land-collected coral sand).   Elegant research by Dr. Halstead and others has shown that the chemical and biological actions of deuterium with organic molecules (body chemicals) may be quite unique. The element deuterium may bond with certain enzymes in a manner that is more stable than water bonds. There is an indication that these deuterium bonds may result in the enhancement of enzymatic reactions in the body (part of the chemistry of life); and this process may even enhance activity of many medications (drugs). These theories are intriguing and I highly recommend that interested readers refer to Dr. Halstead's book, *Fossil Stony Coral Minerals and their Nutritional Application*, (www.wellnesspublishing.com).

Dr. Halstead's book is an authoritative, early account of the biology of coral remnants and he provides an interesting series of references that are relevant to an understanding of the actions of coral calcium. Such references are not found in other books on the subject of coral calcium. Dr. Halstead was a pioneer of research into chelation therapy and he believed that many minerals in coral calcium are naturally chelated. According to the late Dr. Halstead's writings, these afford advantages for the efficient assimilation of minerals for the body. The word "chelate" comes from a Greek word that refers to the "claw" of a crab or lobster. The elements in question are bound by the "claw," a process of chelation. In technical terms, chelation is the incorporation of a metal ion into a heterocyclic (chemical) ring structure (a "pincer-like" chemical effect). This kind of chemical binding process is described as a "bioinorganic" process. In simple terms, it may make elements more available for use by the body.

To avoid technicalities, one can perceive the chelation process in nature to be one of the important processes by which living organisms use metals. In brief, when minerals are chelated they are believed to be more effectively absorbed and utilized by living organisms. Thus, the presence of metals in coral calcium in a chelated format may be another key to the understanding of the benefits of coral calcium as a mineral supplement.

A CLASH OF OPINIONS ON CORAL CALCIUM

Differing opinions on the ideal form of coral minerals to use as a dietary supplement have emerged and re-emerged on a perpetual basis. On the one hand, the late Bruce Halstead MD believed that only coral collected above sea level should be used for human consumption. Dr. Halstead has made compelling arguments that fossilized stony minerals that reached land deposits many thousands of years ago contain bioactive chelated minerals which do not associate themselves with environmental pollutants. These are the pollutants that have emerged as a consequence of industrial revolutions in modern times. Others have argued to the contrary. Furthermore, Dr. Halstead believes that stony coral minerals exert health benefits as a consequence of their global and specific micronutrient profile, not just as a consequence of the calcium content (or magnesium content) of coral remnants.

On the other hand, Mr. Robert Barefoot and his disciples insist that the health benefits of coral calcium are related to its calcium content. His newfound beliefs in the use of below sea level-collected coral remnants, which have an alleged natural 2:1 balance of calcium to magnesium are widely touted. However, Mr. Barefoot once operated in a business promoting land coral and in another business as a spokesman for selling coral calcium in teabags. The origin of the words "coral calcium" is unclear. **I reiterate that the dietary supplement known as coral calcium appears to have much more to do with holistic micronutrient profiles in terms of its biological actions rather than just exerting a benefit through its content of calcium alone.**

The variability in opinions concerning the best type of coral calcium to use are clouded further by propaganda, emerging opinions to support different brands of coral calcium and major uncertainties about how coral calcium may work to provide a health benefit. The principal hypotheses that I propose to explain the biomedical or biochemical actions of coral calcium include:

- **calcium content alone (a rejected concept by many)**
- **balanced calcium and magnesium content (a partial advantage?)**
- **holistic mineral and elemental composition providing micronutrients (likely)**
- **specific micronutrient metals (likely)**
- **specific micronutrient elements e.g., deuterium (plausible)**
- **alterations of body pH with a shift towards alkalinity (naïve component?)**
- **partial provision of a healthy balanced mineral intake (likely)**
- **homeopathic activity (plausible)**
- **Cell Salt Theory proposed initially by Dr. W. H. Schuessler (plausible)**
- **the independent benefits of alkaline ionized water (Coral Calcium Water™, Coralyte™) (www.naturesbenefit.com)?**
- **polarity, electromagnetism of food due to positive mineral elements (questioned)**

I emphasize that the mechanism of action of coral calcium as a dietary supplement remains in question. The possibility that coral calcium exerts a benefit by a homeopathic mechanism or the biochemical expansion of homeopathic theory by Dr. W. H. Schuessler (biochemic theory of "cell salts") are my personal suggestions and represent hypotheses that I believe to be worthy of closer debate and examination. Even if coral calcium is shown to fulfill any therapeutic promise, the mechanism of these putative benefits may remain unclear.

CORAL CALCIUM AND HOMEOPATHY

Marine products (fish, seaweed, coral, etc.) have a long history of use in homeopathic medicines. However, the origin of these homeopathic medical ingredients is difficult to trace. Salts or minerals are frequent inclusions in a large proportion of the many thousands of homeopathic formulae used to treat a wide variety of illnesses (see Boericke's *Materia Medica*). Homeopathic medicine was founded in the 18th century by the celebrated physician Samuel Hahnemann. It was Dr. Hahnemann who reported great health significance and benefits, related to the use of mineral substances in minute amounts in homeopathic remedies. Several physicians have extended Dr. Hahnemann's original concepts of homeopathy. It was Dr. W. H. Schuessler (a renowned German physician) who extended standard homeopathic concepts to a system which he called "biochemistry" (biochemic), with an emphasis on this term representing "the chemistry of life".

In 1880 Dr. Schuessler published a book called *Twelve Tissue Remedies* (a translated title). His treatment methods were not strictly examples of homeopathic treatments. He used 12 cell salts in his treatments, which have been variably described as biochemic salts, tissues remedies, colloids or simply "cell salts". These cell salts were considered by Dr. Schuessler to be essential for normal body function, and he believed in a concept of restoration of vitality and balance to the body. These are not strictly homeopathic concepts, which involve typically the principal of "like healing like" (*similia similibus curantur*). Dr. Schuessler believed that he was supplying the exact constituents that cells were lacking for their normal biochemical functions, not just supplying "homeopathic healing."

Dr. Schuessler went further in his hypotheses. He was interested in astrology and linked each of the 12 cell salts with an astrological marker. These extensions of Schuessler's reasonings did more harm than good when it came to an acceptance of his hypotheses among his colleagues. In brief, the 12 Schuessler cell salts are:

-Silicea (Sagittarius)   - Kali sulphuricum (Virgo)
-Ferrum phosphoricum (Pisces)   - Calcarea sulphuricum (Scorpio)
-Natrum phosphorium (Libra)   - Natrum muriaticum (Aquarius)
-Kali phosphoricum (Aries)   - Kali muriaticum (Gemini)
-Natrum sulphuricum (Taurus)   - Calcarea fluoricum (Cancer)
-Calcarea phosphoricum (Capricorn) - Magnesia phosphoricum (Leo).

While Dr. Schuessler's 12 cell salts may be variably present in material like coral sand and or seawater sediments, there are major differences in elemental profiles between Schuessler's salts and coral calcium. However, Dr. Schuessler "potentized" his salts (a homeopathic technique). I find his hypotheses quite consistent with how coral calcium could work, but not all homeopathic or other physicians believe in this "biochemic system" of treatment. I cannot comment on Schuessler's astrological projections.

Several noted physicians have subscribed to Schuesslers' hypotheses. One proponent was James H. Stephenson MD who died in 1985. Dr. Stephenson was a graduate of Cornell University. He became very interested in astrology and Schuessler's cell salts. Dr. Stephenson was mentored by the homeopathic expert, Elisabeth Wright Hubbard. Ms Hubbard had used Schuessler's salts to cure Dr. Stephenson of chronic pain that he had developed while he was a prisoner of war. In addition, the Australian homeopath, Dr. M. Blackmore, extended and popularized Schuessler's work in his book *Celloids: A Textbook for Physicians* (1958). Dr. Blackmore claimed that he had "refined" Schuessler's cell salt remedies by adding more substantial amounts and ranges of salts (except sodium chloride). Thus, Dr. Blackmore's concepts are even more in keeping with the use of holistic mineral supplements like coral calcium.

OBSERVATIONS ON 12 "MAGIC" HEALING SALTS

The most interesting, popular account of the application of Schuessler's remedies is to be found in the book *Nature's 12 Magic Healers: The Amazing Secrets of Cell Salts*, by Lionel Rolfe and Nigey Lennon (Parker Publishing Company Inc., West Nyack, New York, 1978, reprinted and partially revised by Keats Publishing). In this book, two eminent homeopathic physicians, J. H. Renner MD and William E. S. Jackson MD, comment on the value of Schuessler's cell salts. Dr. Kenner writes in a foreword, *"Tissue salts are not a new, untried discovery. As a medical doctor with over 50 years of experience, I have used these tissue salts with results equal to those documented earlier. In these past 200 years, results have been just fabulous."*

Dr. Schuessler's reasoning and that of his apprentices may raise the eyebrows of the modern-day allopathic (conventional) physician, but Dr. Schuessler's system of cell salt therapies is widely practiced (in modified formats) in many countries, especially Germany. Dr. Schuessler reasoned that when a human cell is reduced to ashes, presumably by heat, there are only 12 minerals left. These 12 minerals were termed "cell salts," but there are more than 12 cell salts present. The reason for Dr. Schuessler's underestimate of the number of cell salts may have been related to limitations in his own laboratory analyses of tissue combustions. Intuitively, Dr. Schuessler and his followers stated that a lack of basic cell salts will prevent nutrients entering cells to provide nourishment, with the result that normal body structure and function is not maintained and disease occurs. **Dr. Schuessler proposed that lack of key cell salts in human diets created major imbalances in the body** and interrupted what Dr. Claude Bernard (the famous French physiologist) had called "The Harmony of Life".

MISUNDERSTOOD HISTORIC PERSPECTIVES ON MINERALS?

Some promoters of coral calcium support their "gobbledygook" claims by misinterpretations of reality, or an inaccurate rehash of early thoughts on natural cures. For the scholarly reader, I refer to work by pioneers of natural medicine such as Henry Lindlahr MD, Charles de Coti-Marsh MD, Wilhelm Heinrich Schuessler MD and others. Each of these revered proponents of natural medicine have stressed the value of minerals in the diet.

It seems increasingly clear that the writings of these early proponents of "natural cures" have been thoughtfully updated in some circumstances, e.g. Dr. Jocelyn Proby's revisions to the works of Dr. Henry Lindlahr MD, but in other contemporary settings, the

work of these earlier supporters of "natural" cures has been bas-
tardized. In some cases, earlier naive notions expressed by "natural
healers" have been replaced by advances in scientific knowledge, but
some redundant notions remain held by some individuals who market coral calcium supplements.

Dr. Lindlahr MD (Natural Therapeutics, Vol. 3, Dietetics,
1914) placed great emphasis on the value of mineral intake for health
and proposed that health begins in the soil. Dr. Jocelyn Proby D.O.
indicates that Dr. Lindlahr got ideas about minerals depletion of soil
and poor health from the work of Dr. Julius Hensel in the late 19th
century. In the early part of the 20th century, Dr. Lindlahr rejected
the value of food on its calorie content alone and proposed that food
value was more related to the provision of essential materials for the
building and repair of tissues (information cited by J. Proby in
Natural Therapeutics by H. Lindlahr). Thus, Dr. Lindlahr was
addressing the "nutrient density" of food – a concept proposed by the
contemporary anti-aging expert Roy Walford MD (Walford, 1986).

Dr. Lindlahr preferred the use of terms such as "Life-
Elements" rather than vitamins and this revolutionary concept, in
1914, drew attention to the essential nature of minerals. In this
early work, there were references to magnetic influences of food and
the generation of positive electricity, which Dr. Lindlahr suggested
was a function of an abundance of positive mineral elements in the
diet. **The primary concept proposed by Lindlahr was that "health
is positive and disease is negative."** These concepts deserve further
analysis and reappraisal, but they are oversimplifications of some
natural therapies to which the more desperate or misinformed may
cling.

Dr. Lindlahr described the functions of food and drinks in
"the economy of the body" in a novel manner. His five food groups
(Groups 1-5) of (1) starches, (2) sugars, (3) fats (oils), (4) proteins
and (5) positive mineral elements (including vitamins or life elements) are relevant to modern theories of how organic-based or
inorganic-based mineral supplements may be valuable for health.

The Group 5 of food types described by Lindlahr included
all dietary inclusions that were low in acid-forming foods that are
found in groups 1-4. This Group 5 was high in positive alkaline
mineral elements including iron, sodium, lime (calcium carbonate
and hydroxide), potassium, magnesium and manganese. It was pro-

posed that these positive minerals could bind acid and even "neutralize or eliminate "morbid materials" from the body. These proposals may be partially correct, but they have not been embraced by modern allopathic medicine. The idea of alkaline elements binding acids in the body is quite naïve. Any effects that alkaline elements have on body pH are indirect effects, exerted through the complex acid-alkali buffering systems of the body.

Dr. Lindlahr was somewhat critical of the use of "cell salts", as proposed by Dr. Wilhelm Schuessler, because of their inorganic nature, but he did acknowledge their potential usefulness. The debate on whether or not inorganic sources of minerals (rocks) are as health-giving as organic sources of minerals (vegetables or fruit juices) continues today. Alternative thinking physicians believe mainly in organic sources of minerals and coral calcium may provide one of the best origins for a holistic mineral supplement because of its birth (origination) in living coral (organic sources of the microelements).

The matters that I discuss have been summarized by Jocelyn Proby DO in her revisions and additions to the work of Dr. Henry Lindlahr MD (*Philosophy of Natural Therapeutics*, C.W. Daniel Company Ltd, Walden, UK, 1914). Dr. Proby states in 1975:

"Lindlahr (referring to Dr. Henry Lindlahr writing in his book entitled "Philosophy of Natural Therapeutics", 1914) does here admit a certain usefulness in the Schuessler tissue salts, but he is not keen on them because of their "inorganic" character. His disciple, Mackinnon, on the other hand, looked on them with much more favor. These salts as originally prepared and advocated by Schuessler do seem to be something of a mystery in that while they appear to be intended as dietary supplements which are given to make up deficiencies or to correct imbalances, they are in fact prepared after the manner of homeopathic remedies which normally act in the body in accordance with the law of similars. It would appear very doubtful whether the amount of the minerals contained in them could in fact be sufficient to make up deficiencies in the chemical sense. It would seem more likely that the effects which they undoubtedly have are produced rather by causing a change in body metabolism which normalizes that metabolism in specific ways. It this is so, there can be little objection to them on the grounds of their "inorganic" character. More recently there has grown a school of

Biochemic Therapy associated, in England at least, with the name of Dr. Gilbert. This school absolutely denies that there is any essential difference in the case of mineral substances which are required by the body between those derived from animal or vegetable tissue and those derived from inorganic sources. They prepare such minerals from inorganic sources and use them in sufficient quantities to correct deficiencies and imbalances which they believe to exist. Such biochemic food supplements are usually prepared by an elaborate process of trituration but they are not potentized in the same way as homeopathic remedies or the Schuessler salts. It is claimed that not only are they harmless but that they are, in many cases, more easily assimilated and used by the body than the same substances taken in vegetable or fresh foods. There is here a definite conflict of opinion but it may be that there is some element of truth in both points of view though they may at first appear irreconcilable. It does seem that the body is intended to get the mineral substances it needs from food, and Julius Hensel who was the first great exponent of biochemic ideas believed that health must begin in the soil and that the health of the soil and crops must be maintained not by chemical fertilizers but by putting back into the soil what has been taken from it. This he did largely by the use of ground rocks as well as animal and vegetable residues and manures. Others have done the same thing by the use of seaweed in various forms. On the other hand, it does appear that the body has a certain limited ability to assimilate and use mineral substances more directly either from water or from such substances as common salt and, if Hensel and some of his followers are right, in the form of ground rocks. It is surely not impossible that there is a real difference between minerals derived from vegetable or animal tissues and those derived directly from water or rocks, even though this difference may not be detectable by ordinary chemical analysis. On the other hand, it may be that certain ways of preparing mineral substances by great refinement or grinding may enable them to be used directly by the body in a very effective and rapid manner....

CALCIUM INTAKE: MULTIPLE BENEFITS

There are several recognized health benefits of calcium supplementation, other than the obvious effects of maintaining healthy teeth and bones. Calcium has been demonstrated to have a mild anti-hypertensive (blood-pressure lowering) effect. In double-blind crossover studies, people with moderate hypertension who received 1 gram per day of calcium for eight weeks had reductions in blood pressure during calcium administration. Later, I review the predictable mild blood pressure-lowering ability of coral calcium that has been observed in small scale, open label studies in Japan.

Reductions in blood lipids, including cholesterol and triglycerides, have been observed in short- and long-term studies of calcium supplementation, thereby giving calcium a potential role in the promotion of cardiovascular wellness. Adequate calcium intake is known to play a valuable role in the prevention of cancer, especially colon cancer. It appears that calcium in the diet can prevent the recurrence of colon polyps. Polyps are pre-cancerous growths in the large bowel. Furthermore, calcium deficiency has been associated with many other diseases. However, the amount of calcium required to achieve these effects may be different from the amount of calcium that is present in coral calcium. Thus, the notion of the "calcium factor" when explaining the actions of coral calcium is further in question.

HEALTHY BONES; CLEAR BENEFITS FROM CALCIUM AND OTHER MINERALS

The beneficial effects of calcium supplementation on bone density and bone loss in pre-menopausal and postmenopausal women are well recognized. Several studies in Western society have shown that women have a loss of bone density when they have a daily calcium consumption of less than 400 mg/day. Loss of bone density tends to be much less in women who have a calcium intake of approximately 750mg/day or more. Even though some scientific studies have failed to show a major beneficial effect of calcium supplementation in preventing or reversing osteoporosis, **an overwhelming body of opinion is in favor of calcium supplementation as a preventive and treatment measure for osteoporosis.** (See the book, "The Antiporosis Plan", by S. Holt, www.wellnesspublishing.com).

AMOUNTS AND TYPES OF DIETARY CALCIUM

Accepting the importance of dietary calcium supplementation, the amount and chemical type of calcium and the source and
format of calcium in the diet are believed to be important variables
in the promotion of bone health and general well-being. Calcium
carbonate is the most frequently used salt of calcium in dietary supplement preparations and calcium is present as carbonate in coral
calcium. However, experts believe that the natural origin of calcium
in coral calcium (or other natural sources of calcium e.g. egg-shell
calcium) presents advantages (see Dr. Halstead's hypotheses about
chelation and coral calcium). Calcium supplements should be taken
shortly before meals or with food to provide optimal absorption
into the body. Contrary to popular belief, relatively insoluble salts
of calcium, such as calcium carbonate, can be absorbed in the relative absence of gastric acid; even though absorption is less efficient.

I believe that an optimal amount of calcium to be taken in the
diet of most people is 800 – 1000 mg/day for average adults and
about 1-2g/day for young, mature and elderly adults. Several studies
have indicated that calcium intake in many diets may often be below
the RDA (RDI), especially in the elderly. Only about one quarter of
all children of school age receive an optimum amount of calcium in
their diets. **The ideal way to supplement calcium in the diet is to eat
calcium-rich foods, but the range of such foods is limited in "average" diets and dietary supplements represent a convenient and consistent source of calcium (see www.naturesbenefit.com).** There are
several adverse effects of taking too much calcium in the diet, especially if an individual is not healthy and if renal (kidney) failure is present. However, there is some emerging evidence that taking calcium
from natural sources (e.g. coral calcium and eggshell calcium) may
lead to less adverse effects such as high or low blood calcium levels
(hypercalcemia and hypocalcemic, see www.antiporosis.com and
www.naturesbenefit.com), but such evidence is arguable.

REVISITING CALCIUM SUPPLEMENTS

An increased intake of calcium from calcium-rich foods is
required by many people, including those individuals taking coral
calcium at current recommended daily intakes of 1.5 g/day (1500

mg of coral calcium). **Increasing calcium intake is often a difficult feat for many people on an average American diet.** A list of calcium-rich foods is shown in Table 10.

CALCIUM

FOOD	AMOUNT	CONTENT (mg)
Sardines with bones	_ cup	500
Mackerel with bones	_ cup	300
Milk	1 cup	288
Fortified rice milk	1 cup	280
Broccoli	1 cup	178
Mustard greens, cooked	1 cup	180
Canned red salmon	_ cup	275
Fortified soy milk	1 cup	280
Cooked brown rice	1 cup	20
Cooked oats	1 cup	40
Lentils	1 cup	50
Black beans	1 cup	60
Walnuts	_ cup	70
Hazelnuts	_ cup	115
Soybeans	1 cup	130
Tofu	1 cup	150
Lima beans	1 cup	60
Alfalfa sprouts	1 cup	25
Romaine lettuce	1 cup	40
Almonds	_ cup	.175

Table 10: A list of calcium-containing foods with their approximate calcium content. Please note that the calcium absorption from these different foods may vary considerably. Foods may be better listed in terms of calcium content that is available for use by the body.

The emphasis placed by some nutritionists on milk and dairy products as a good source of calcium requires cautious interpretation. Whole milk and dairy products contain unwanted calories with a high content of saturated fat and cholesterol. Furthermore, milk protein allergies are a significant issue. It is notable that several scientists have highlighted the potential of food allergies (e.g. milk protein allergy) as a potential cause of osteoporosis, and other chronic diseases, but this is arguable. Milk protein allergy has been indirectly associated with asthma and asthma is associated with osteoporosis (www.antiporosis.com). There are several reasons why people may want to avoid milk as their primary, dietary source of calcium.

EXAMINING OTHER DIETARY SUPPLEMENT SOURCES OF CALCIUM

There has been much debate about the ideal form of calcium supplement and Table 11 addresses some advantages and limitations of several forms of calcium that are used as dietary supplements.

Type of Calcium	Concentration Calcium	Advantages	Disadvantages
Microcrystalline Hydroxyapatite	25%	Well absorbed complete bone food, absorbed by those with poor digestion	Costly source for elemental calcium, may contain toxic heavy metals
Citrate	24%	Well absorbed, may reduce the risk of kidney stones	A lot needs to be used in a supplement because of low calcium concentration
Di-Calcium Phosphate Calcium Concentration	28%	Advantage of calcium to phosphorus ratio. inexpensive form of elemental calcium	Not well absorbed in patients with high dietary phosphorus intakes, may further distort normal calcium to phosphorus levels
Lactate	15%	Well absorbed. Expensive source of elemental calcium	May contain allergens, e.g. yeast and milk protein from fermentation processes.

Carbonate	40%	Least expensive form of calcium, highest content of elemental calcium	Variable absorption, may create gastric distress (switches on acid secretion calcium in stomach and causes constipation)
Bone Meal	39%	Complete bone food. Rich source of elemental calcium	May contain toxic levels of lead, arsenic, and cadmium. Organic constituents are destroyed in processing
Coral Calcium	24-42%	More than calcium, up to 70 micronutrient minerals. Best taken in ratio of 2:1 calcium to magnesium. No tendency to cause hyper-calcemia	Cost, but it is more than just a calcium supplement
Eggshell Calcium (Natures Calcium™)	35-40%	A very attractive form of calcium supplement, well absorbed and inexpensive. Reduced tendency to cause hypercalcemia	None

Table 11: Types of calcium supplements: advantages and disadvantages.

While much debate has occurred about the best form of calcium to take as a supplement, many advantages have been proposed for forms of calcium from natural sources. These forms of calcium produced by living organisms have been particularly favored. Exciting new options involve the use of calcium from coral remnants (coral calcium) and the use of calcium from eggshells (www.naturescalcium.com, www.ovocal.com, www.naturesbenefit.com, www.antiporosis.com).

CHAPTER SUMMARY

The potential mechanisms of action of coral calcium are legion. More is unknown than is known on the subject of coral calcium. Coral calcium is more than just a "calcium supplement". Its biological effects of potential health benefits remain uncharted and the mechanisms of these benefits are the subject of much debate and the need for initial speculation with much further research.

CORAL CALCIUM IS A HOLISTIC SOURCE
OF MINERALS

CHAPTER 6:

EMERGING SCIENCE AND LONGEVITY

SCIENTIFIC STUDIES OF CORAL CALCIUM

Studies performed at the University of Ryukyus and the University of Okinawa have shown that calcium absorption from coral calcium into the body of experimental animals was better than absorption of calcium from milk-associated-calcium and cow bone-derived calcium, or hydroxyapatite, (see Table 12). These feeding experiments in animals were carefully controlled and the organs and blood of the animals were analyzed for calcium and magnesium contents. An incidental finding in these studies was a favorable change in blood cholesterol. This type of coral calcium has been used in the products Barefoot Coral Calcium Plus™, and Marine Coral Minerals™ in 1.5 gram daily amounts. **Assertions that calcium is 100% absorbed from coral calcium are frankly untrue.**

UNFORTUNATELY, CONTROLLED CLINICAL TRIALS ON THE TREATMENT BENEFITS OF CORAL CALCIUM DO NOT EXIST

	Control Group	Coral Minerals	Milk	Cow Bone
Calcium (Ca)				
Intake (mg/3 days)	319.3 +/- 13.9	360.2 +/- 6.3	313.2 +/- 6.4	318.9 +/- 15.4
Absorption (mg/3 days)	177.8 +/- 7.7	251.6 +/- 15.1	195.3 +/- 7.0	213.8 +/- 12.8
Percent (%) Absorption	55.9 +/- 2.1	69.6 +/- 3.1	62.4 +/- 1.8	66.9 +/- 1.4
Magnesium (Mg)				
Intake (mg/3 days)	131.0 +/- 5.7	161.8 +/- 2.8	131.2 +/- 2.7	161.7 +/- 7.8
Absorption (mg/3 days)	70.1 +/- 3.4	117.9 +/- 5.0	66.6 +/- 4.3	109.6 +/- 6.4
Percent (%) Absorption	53.6 +/- 1.6	72.8 +/- 2.3	50.8 +/- 3.2	69.7 +/- 1.8
Phosphorus (P)				
Intake (mg/3 days)	278.3 +/- 12.1	316.8 +/- 5.5	279.3 +/- 7.3	273.2 +/- 13.2
Absorption (mg/3 days)	197.6 +/- 8.2	267.7 +/- 6.9	192.1 +/- 3.4	177.7 +/- 9.5
Percent (%) Absorption	71.1 +/- 1.5	84.5 +/- 1.1	68.8 +/- 1.1	65.2 +/- 2.9

Table 12: The absorption of calcium from coral calcium in these animal experiments was superior to the absorption of calcium from several other forms of calcium supplements. Calcium, magnesium and phosphorus absorption rates are shown.

GYRATING BLOOD CALCIUM LEVELS

Two Japanese researchers (S. Kawamura and T. Taniuchi) have written an illuminating account of the use of calcium supplements, including coral calcium, in their book, *Warning! Calcium Deficiency* (Shundaiyoyosha Publishing Co., Tokyo, Japan, 1999). These researchers reported a 30-year study with 20,000 case histories concerning more than 40 different, over-the-counter calcium supplements. They found that people taking large amounts of ionized calcium often experienced adverse symptoms due to high blood calcium levels (hypercalcemia). They noted that rapid swings in blood calcium could occur with occasional abrupt lowering of blood calcium in individuals taking calcium supplements (hypocalcemia). These Japanese scientists found that individuals who took coral calcium or other marine calcium products did not tend to suffer from states of high or low blood calcium. The lack of gyration of blood calcium when taking coral calcium is a real advantage, according to the aforementioned Japanese scientists (cited by R. Barefoot in "Barefoot on Coral Calcium: An Elixir of Life").

CALCIUM ABSORPTION FROM FOOD ENRICHED WITH CORAL CALCIUM

In 1999, Dr. Kunihiko Ishitani and colleagues reported the superior absorption of calcium from the intake of coral calcium added to food (*J. Nutr. Sci. Vitaminol.*, 45, 509-517, 1999). In this small, but well-controlled study, these Japanese researchers used crackers containing coral calcium powder and compared them with plain calcium carbonate containing crackers, in terms of the ability of a small number of subjects (six men and six women) to absorb calcium from the dietary intake of these crackers. In brief, the amount of intestinal absorption of calcium from crackers containing coral calcium (in a form of coral calcium of calcium to magnesium in a ratio of 2:1), was greater than the absorption of calcium from crackers containing only calcium carbonate. There was wide variability in the amount of calcium absorbed in these subjects who participated in the studies, regardless of whether or not coral calcium containing crackers or calcium carbonate containing crackers were eaten.

The authors of this calcium absorption study, using coral calcium, referred to a study by Dr. K. Suzuki and colleagues, (presented in 1997) and referred to previously, as showing enhanced absorption of calcium in rats from coral calcium in comparison with a number of other forms of calcium (Suzuki K et al, Calcium utilization from natural coral calcium – A coral preparation with a calcium-magnesium content ratio of 2:1. Abstracts of Papers Presented at the 44th Jpn. Soc. Nutr. Betterment, p. 145, Fukuoka, Japan). The authors of these two absorption studies imply that the shallow seas around the Ryukyus Islands of Okinawa may yield coral sand with approximately 20% and 10% calcium and magnesium content, respectively. Recall, the vehement arguments to the contrary by some suppliers of bulk coral calcium.

CORAL CALCIUM AND OSTEOPOROSIS

Scientific studies performed at the Futaba Nutrition School of the Kagawa Nutrition University in Japan show the benefit of coral calcium in improvements in bone mineral density, when coral calcium is given in a balanced composition of 600 mg of calcium with 300 mg of magnesium (calcium:magnesium, 2:1 ratio). This research study was presented at the 52nd Japanese Society of Nutrition and Food Science (April, 1998). In this well-conducted study, there were six experimental groups of subjects. These groups were:

1. A group receiving coral calcium and low-fat milk as calcium reinforcement in the diet.
2. A group taking the same calcium reinforcement in the diet with exercise in first period of study in the form of strength training and in the third period walking.
3. A group taking the same calcium reinforcement with exercise in the first period as walking and in the third period as strength training.
4. A group engaged in exercise only as in 2 above.
5. A group engaged in exercise only as in 3 above.
6. A control group.

These studies show that all active experimental groups, except the control group, showed increases in bone mineral density. The greatest change in bone mineral density was shown in group 2, who took calcium reinforcement with milk and coral calcium, together with exercise consisting of initial strength training, followed later in the study by walking. This study is highly relevant to the fundamental components of products that use coral calcium to build bone density (see *"The Antiporosis Plan"* by Stephen Holt MD, www.wellnesspublishing.com). The dietary supplement product Antiporosis™ uses a unique form of calcium supplementation with a combination of coral calcium and eggshell calcium (Natures Calcium™). *The Antiporosis Plan* recommends nutrition and lifestyle change, (especially exercise) for the management of osteoporosis (www.naturesbenefit.com and www.antiporosis.com).

I do not believe that coral calcium supplements alone are adequate for the nutritional management of osteoporosis. Current recommended intake of coral calcium supplements do not come close to the RDI of calcium, perhaps with the exception of Coral Calcium Powder™ (in a dosage of 3g/day) produced by Natures Benefit Inc. (www.naturesbenefit.com).

RETURNING TO THE IMPORTANCE OF VITAMIN D

The biochemistry of vitamin D is very complex. Calcium works together with vitamin D (especially vitamin D3) and neither nutrient can be effective without each other. A substantial proportion of calcium absorption into the body (about 30%) is under the control of vitamin D3. Also, this vitamin exerts major influences on calcium metabolism by the body. While some controversy has existed concerning the bone-building actions of calcium and vitamin D in individuals with osteoporosis, many scientific studies point to the benefits of this vital combination of nutrients, especially in senile (or elderly-type) osteoporosis.

When the levels of vitamin D are inadequate or fall in the body, the blood levels of calcium will tend to fall and calcium cannot be laid down in bone. A deficiency of vitamin D causes a specific bone disease called osteomalacia (rickets), where there is insufficient calcium in bones, making them rubbery and weak. This disorder is a different disease than osteoporosis. Rickets can cause many skeletal deformities (e.g., bumps on bones, bow-legs). The disease of rickets has been largely eradicated in Western countries by fortification of foods (especially milk) with vitamin D.

Vitamin D is synthesized in the body as a consequence of exposure to sunlight (an ultimate "nutrient"). A lack of exposure to sunshine made the disease of rickets a particular problem in several groups of people (e.g. underground workers, coal miners, the elderly who are housebound etc.). Vitamin D deficiency plays a major role in senile osteoporosis, which is quite often responsive to vitamin D administration and adequate, but safe, exposure to sunlight.

Deficiencies of vitamin D will cause bone to lose calcium because falling blood levels of calcium results in calcium being taken from the "calcium bank" in bones. The recommended daily intake of vitamin D is 400 international units, but several studies have shown advantages of extra vitamin D in certain groups of individuals. However, vitamin D is toxic when taken in excess. Vitamin D is a major component of *The Antiporosis Plan* to combat osteo-porosis. When vitamin D is taken in appropriate doses in combination with calcium and other bone-building nutrients, it is highly beneficial for individuals wishing to prevent or engage the nutritional management of osteoporosis (www.antiporosis.com). **Recent advice from coral calcium promoters to engage in extended, unprotected sunlight exposure is dangerous, as are their recommendations to take toxic amounts of vitamin D.**

THE SUNLIGHT SAGA

Vitamin D is active in its D3 form which is synthesized in the skin as a consequence of sunlight. On the one hand, moderate sunlight exposure is necessary for vitamin D synthesis, but on the other hand, modern science has clearly defined the health risks of over-exposure to sunlight. I reiterate that recommendations by some individuals that hours of unprotected sun exposure is health-giving must be considered nonsense.

Medical science has recorded that factors that limit exposure to sunlight are useful in the prevention of premature skin aging and cancer. However, gross lack of exposure to the sun can diminish the body status of vitamin D and may secondarily exert a negative effect on bone health. Healthy exposure to sunlight should be controlled exposure which will meet most of the body's vitamin D requirement, in most climates, in most people. It appears that it is only the elderly in Western communities that may be at risk of vitamin D deficiency due to a lack of sunlight exposure.

MORE ON MAGNESIUM

The role of magnesium in the support of bone structure and function has been grossly underestimated. **More than one half of all of the body's magnesium is found in bone tissue.** Magnesium exerts multiple effects on body chemistry and it controls bone health. A deficiency of magnesium may result in a tissue resistance to the actions of vitamin D3 and parathyroid hormone; and it may cause an interference with the release of parathyroid hormone. Despite the known importance of magnesium for bone health, there have been relatively few studies on the ability of magnesium supplements to increase bone density in people with osteoporosis, or other chronic diseases.

Magnesium has many beneficial effects on cardiovascular function and it is an important enzyme co-factor. In one important reported study in people with malabsorption due to celiac disease (a sensitivity to gluten from wheat, a food allergy), magnesium supplements were shown to improve blood levels of parathyroid hormone and cause increases in bone density. The higher magnesium content of certain forms of coral calcium or the addition of magnesium salts to coral calcium may have some advantages (vide infra).

MAGNESIUM DEPLETION

Recent studies suggest that magnesium is often depleted from fruits and vegetables, especially when artificial fertilizers are used. For example, the magnesium content of spinach cultivated by organic farming is recorded at an average of about 100 mg per 100 grams, whereas with the use of agricultural chemicals the average content of magnesium is about 70 mg per 100 grams (about 30% less). Even washing and cutting vegetables may deplete magnesium content by a factor of up to one half.

There are many causes of magnesium deficiency in humans. These include low dietary intake of magnesium, poor soil mineral content, food processing, alcohol intake, smoking, physical exercise and mental stress. The special role of magnesium and calcium balance in cardiovascular health was illustrated in studies of deaths from ischemic heart disease. The ratio of dietary intake of calcium to magnesium seems to be quite important for cardiovascular health (Figure 2). Scientific studies imply that dietary intakes of calcium to magnesium in a ratio of higher than 2:1 may increase deaths from ischemic heart disease (Figure 2).

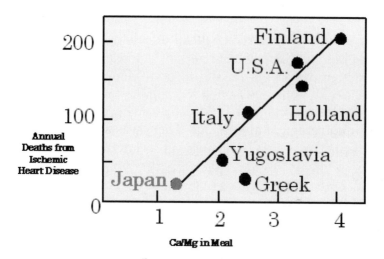

Figure 2: Death rates per 100,000 increase in nations that have a high ratio of calcium-to-magnesium intake. The ratio of calcium to magnesium of no more than 2:1 seems often to be optimal. Note that these are epidemiological observations, and factors other than the ratio of calcium to magnesium in the diet contribute to deaths from coronary heart disease (Data from Karppanen, et al, 1960). Please note that these data imply that low ratios of Ca:Mg exist in Japanese diets.

Some scientists have concluded that a calcium to magnesium ratio of 2:1 is the ideal ratio of intake of these elements in the diet. Furthermore, several Japanese scientists have indicated that coral calcium with this natural balance of calcium to magnesium of 2:1 is an ideal dietary source of these elements (www.naturesbenefit.com); but the data could be interpreted as showing an advantage for a ratio of Ca:Mg in the diet of much less than 2:1.

EMERGING CLINICAL SCIENCE ON CORAL CALCIUM

Recent open-label clinical trials of coral calcium in individuals with a variety of common diseases have been presented by K. Ishitani MD, of Higashi Sapporo Hospital (data on file Marine Bio Co Ltd. and Natures Benefit Inc). Dr. Ishitani and his colleagues have administered 2.8 g of balanced (Ca: Mg, 2:1 ratio) coral calcium to more than 20 patients for a period of three months. These researchers observed alterations in bone density, blood lipids and blood pressure together with alterations in symptoms such as headache, heart palpitations, peripheral edema (limb swelling) and emotional status, including measures of anger, anxiety and muscle spasm. Overall, Dr. Ishitani described very favorable effects from the administration of coral calcium in these subjects. Blood pressure was reduced from average of 140 to 132 mm Hg and total cholesterol fell by an average of about 7%. There was a tendency for blood lipids to alter favorably, with a rise in serum HDL and a fall in triglycerides. Some inconsistent benefits were observed in emotional state and reduction in heart palpitations. These data are fascinating but they are incomplete; and they may be explained in part by the benefits of multi-mineral supplementation.

CORAL CALCIUM AND BRAIN FUNCTION

Coral calcium-treated water was administered in a dose of 1.5 g approximately to 12 students by Dr. S.Sugimoto of Aichi Syukutoku University, Japan and indirect measurements of central nervous system function were made by electroencephalogram (EEG). There was a measurable increase in total alpha-1 wave activity on an EEG when the coral-treated water was given to the students, compared with the administration of regular tap water. The alpha-2 wave activity in the brain was also increased by the administration of coral water. These results imply that coral calcium may have a stabilizing effect on the CNS with a tendency to "relaxation" (data on file Natures Benefit Inc, provided by Marine Bio Co Ltd). The potential "relaxing" actions of calcium and magnesium are well described in popular alternative medicine literature.

CORAL CALCIUM AND BLOOD SUGAR

In recent experiments (2002), Dr. Ishitani has studied a small group of patients with diabetes mellitus who received 2.8 g of coral calcium with a lower content of magnesium (Ca: Mg, 15:1 ratio). Over a three-month period, Dr. Ishitani showed improvements in blood sugar control in two of four patients with diabetes mellitus, but the numbers of subjects studied (n = 4) do not permit statistical evaluations. There are several reasons why coral calcium could improve blood sugar control in diabetics including the observations (in vivo and in vitro) that a ratio of calcium to magnesium of approximately 17:1 is optimal for insulin production. Calcium alone promotes insulin production and magnesium activates insulin receptors. Much more research is required to further define the role of mineral replacement in diabetic control.

CORAL CALCIUM AS A DIGESTIVE AID

Some new observations involve the study of coral calcium as an antiacid by the novel incorporation of coral calcium into chewing gum, or used as a suspension. Dr. M. Mori MD of the Institute of Clinical and Pharmacokinetic Study, Japan, studied nine patients with heartburn and eight patients with non specific abdominal complaints. In these studies, all nine patients with heartburn had complete symptomatic improvement and 25% of those with non-specific digestive complaints completely improved, whereas the remaining eight individuals showed lesser degrees of improvement. Coral calcium appears to exert an acid-neutralizing capability in these experiments (data on file Natures Benefit Inc, provided by Marine Bio Co Ltd).

THE HEALTH BENEFITS OF CORAL CALCIUM

There are now many hundreds (perhaps thousands) of testimonials on the health benefits of coral calcium, but no controlled scientific studies have emerged. Some zealous promoters of supplements believe that coral calcium has panacea benefits for health. Such people are best ignored, at this stage. While I have attempted to pinpoint the mechanism(s) of the health benefits of Okinawan coral calcium material, no single consensus opinion exists. In summary, I favor the notion that coral calcium is a valuable holistic mineral supplement. It has apparent potent and versatile health benefits that require much more research and systematized documentation. The putative benefits of coral calcium are displayed on the Internet by many people, as are the comments of the skeptics. I must advise that readers avoid websites making illegal treatment claims. The quality of their product may be tantamount to their "ill-founded" claims.

THE OKINAWA PROGRAM: STUDYING LONGEVITY

Longevity among Okinawans is striking (Figure 3). The book, *The Okinawa Program* (2000), written by BJ Willcox MD, D Craig Willcox PhD, and Makoto Suzuki MD, describes how Okinawan people may achieve longevity. The celebrated practitioner of alternative medicine, Andrew Weil MD writes his own observations on how Okinawans may enjoy healthy and long life in the foreword to *The Okinawa Program*. Both the authors of this book and Dr. Weil describe the notable differences between the people of Okinawa and the mainland Japanese and Westerners. This book focuses upon many aspects of lifestyle that are known to be associated with health and long life. These factors include a good level of physical activity, and the eating of fish and soy foods, with abundant fruits and vegetables. The social interactions in Okinawa and the sense of community spirit give Okinawan people an apparently greater self-responsibility for their health, according to Dr. Weil.

**LONGEVITY IN OKINAWA, JAPAN MAY BE DUE
TO MORE THAN JUST MINERAL ENRICHMENT
OF THE ENVIRONMENT**

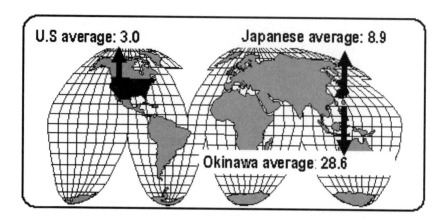

Figure 3: This simple figure reinforces the reports of longevity experienced in Okinawa, Japan.

While the authors stress the importance of vitamin and mineral intake for health, the book entitled "The Okinawa Program" on the longevity of Okinawan people is not focused on the use of coral calcium. However, the research of the Okinawa Program has shown that higher levels of lifelong calcium intake may have occurred in the elite elderly (centenarians in Okinawa). Bradley J. Willcox MD and his colleagues indicate that men and women in Okinawa who have reached centenarian status may obtain about 625 mg and 400 mg of calcium from food, on a respective basis. These scientists do stress that Okinawan people obtain a significant amount of calcium from their drinking water due to the presence of coral deposits on the islands. The authors of *The Okinawa Program* cite the book, *A Professional Handbook of Complementary and Alternative Medicine* (Springhouse Corporation, PA, 1999), as a reference that hip fracture rates are low in Okinawa largely as a consequence of the calcium from coral "deposits" that are present in drinking water in Okinawa.

CORAL CALCIUM, ANTI-AGING AND LONGEVITY

Coral calcium has emerged as an interesting dietary supplement in the category of natural "anti-aging" products. While the link between longevity among Okinawans and coral calcium is not completely clear, there are several lines of reasoning that support an anti-aging role for the dietary, mineral-enriching properties of coral calcium (Halstead, 1999, Barefoot, 2001) or coral calcium-treated water (Willcox et al, 2000).

There are numerous communities throughout the world that enjoy longevity. Roy Walford MD, in his book, *The 120-Year Diet*, describes the long average life span of Hunzas in India and relates this as a potential factor in their drinking of mineral enriched glacial water ("glacial milk"). However, the Hunzas are vegetarians who eat diets rich in health-giving whole grains, vegetables and dietary fiber.

The native Indian populations of Guatemala form an interesting precedent concerning the value of dietary calcium for cardiovascular health. These Indians often have at least 1200 mg of calcium per day (the new US calcium RDI for adults) in their diets, perhaps as a consequence of the use of lime water in the baking of tortillas (Walford, 1986). The benefits of high calcium intake in the diet can be abolished or compromised by other dietary factors. For example, Finland has a high per capita intake of dietary calcium but it is derived mainly from dairy products with a high saturated fat and cholesterol content. Unfortunately, Finland has the highest death rate from heart disease per capita of the population in the world.

There has been much debate about the role of minerals in the health of Okinawans, but I have indicated that the evidence for this is mainly as a consequence of associations or correlations (Holt, 2002 and 2003). Several authors have expressed caution about the value of correlation or testimonial evidence in anti-aging research. Dr. Walford, a renowned anti-aging researcher from UCLA, states, *"Correlation can be seductive, but it's not actual proof."* The documented longevity of Okinawans and their mineral-rich environment has proven very seductive to anti-aging researchers who have started to examine the effects of coral calcium on longevity in animals.

In one experiment performed by Professor N. Tominaga of the Department of Medical Zoology of Saitama Medical School, 22 rats were divided into two groups receiving a similar diet, except one group received normal tap water whereas the other group received alkaline ionized water, prepared by treating tap water with coral calcium. The results, shown in Figure 4, are striking in that the coral water group had, on average, a much longer life span. While this is not proof of a longevity effect of coral calcium in humans (and the results may not be statistically significant), it is very promising data, similar to the kind used by respected anti-aging researchers, such as R.Walford MD.

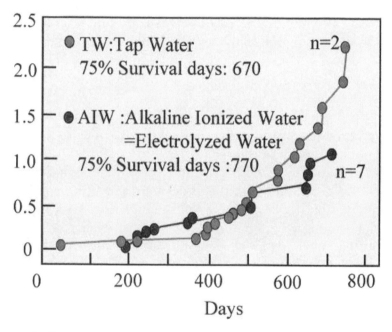

Figure 4: This graph shows enhanced survival in rats that were given alkaline ionized water compared with regular tap water (n = 22 animals, Kaplan-Meier method) (data from Prof. N. Tominaga of the Dept. of Medical Zoology of Saitama Medical School, data on file Natures Benefit Inc., with courtesy of Marine Bio Co. Ltd).

THE WALFORD 120-YEAR DIET

Dr. Walford has reviewed the Okinawan experience of longevity and proposes that this demonstrated life extension is related to the eating of a low-calorie but "nutrient-dense" diet (like "The Walford Diet" or "High/Low Diet"). There are excellent records of dietary patterns and health parameters in Okinawa and other areas of Japan. Okinawa is not only distinguished by the higher average age of its population but also by maximum human survival times—in Okinawa, there are 15 to 37 centenarians per 100,000 of the population. The data presented by Dr. Walford on Okinawan longevity deserves a close look. Dr. Walford argues that the daily caloric intake of Okinawan schoolchildren is about 62% that of the recommended daily caloric intake in Japan. However, the diet is adequate in vitamins and proteins and relatively low in salt and sugar, compared with diets in other locations in Japan. **What does stand out in Okinawa is the enhanced mineral intake in the diet,** a factor not readily acknowledged by Dr. Walford in his discussions of the Okinawan experience.

I believe that Dr. Walford's theories about low-calorie, nutrient-dense diets and longevity are very compelling, and I believe that one important aspect of "nutrient density" of meals that pushes the balance toward longevity is mineral enrichment.

CORAL CALCIUM FOR PETS

While many testimonials emerge on the benefits of coral calcium in humans, a striking number of beneficial reports of the use of coral calcium in beloved companion animals appear on a regular basis. This may not be a surprise as holistic veterinarians report the benefits of adequate calcium and mineral intake in pets. In the leading book on holistic veterinary medicine ("Complementary and Alternative Veterinary Medicine, Principles and Practice," edited by A. Schoen and S. Wynn, Mosby, Times Mirror Publications, St. Louis, Missouri, 1998), experts review the benefits of mineral supplementation in dogs, cats and horses. Body tissues and fluids in dogs, cats and horses contain minerals that are essential to many body structures and functions.

The forms in which mineral supplements are taken appear to be important because of differences in absorption between natural and inert minerals. There is no doubt that some pets may have a dietary deficiency of one or other vital mineral. Minerals have a "macronutrient" or "micronutrient" status. Many breeders and animal experts believe in good nutritional support with minerals in many circumstances. For example, nutritional and mineral requirements increase during phases of the growth of pets, and during times of stress, extra physical activity, illness, old age, and breeding or following gestation.

Calcium and other essential elements are extremely important in animal care. Dr. Shawn Messonnier, D.V. M., an expert on holistic medicine, describes minerals as available in four forms. These forms include inorganic sources, organic sources (e.g. coral calcium), colloidal preparations and crystalloidal minerals. In his book ("Natural Health Bible for Dogs and Cats," Prima Publishing, Prima Pets, S. Messonnier, Roseville, CA, 2001), Dr. Messonnier explains the advantage of organic forms of minerals, such as those found in trace amounts in coral calcium (e.g. selenium, chromium and iron). Dr. Messonnier is cautious about the overuse of "calcium pills", such as inorganic calcium carbonate, but the advantage of coral calcium may be the provision of a holistic profile of mineral elements in very small amounts (parts per million).

The macroelements (calcium, phosphorus, potassium, sodium and magnesium) are all found in coral calcium and these elements are necessary for a healthy bone structure, nerve and muscle function, regulation of pressures in body fluids and the balance of pH in the body. Furthermore, veterinarians have learned that the microminerals (e.g. iron, zinc, copper, manganese, iodine and selenium) are important in enzyme systems in the body that drive the chemistry of life (metalloenzymes). Experts point to the importance of mineral deficiencies as a major cause of metabolic disturbances (unbalanced body chemistry) and growth problems in pets. In fact, these types of deficiencies may often pass unrecognized by owners and pet care givers.

When it comes to pets, coral calcium provides a very interesting mineral profile and the major functions of essential trace elements have been well described in both conventional and alternative veterinary literature. The benefits of supplementing minerals are summarized in Table 13. Table 13 is an adaptation of information published in the book ("Complementary and Alternative Veterinary Medicine, Principles and Practice," edited by A. Schoen and S. Wynn, Mosby, Times Mirror Publications, St. Louis, Missouri, 1998). While clear benefits of correction of deficiencies of mineral intake are apparent in Table 13, one must be aware that excess minerals can cause toxicity. In particular, caution is required with mineral supplementation in pups and kittens. Again, it is important to note that the small content of many trace minerals in coral calcium supplements provide a real advantage of avoiding excessive amounts of minerals that can occur with other types of mineral supplements.

REQUIREMENT (DOG AND CAT)

MINERAL	UNITS	IN DIET*	DEFICIENCY
Calcium	%	0.5†-0.9	Occurs when meat or organ tissues comprise majority of diet; initially: lameness, stiffness, reluctance to move, constipation, enlarged metaphyses, splayed toes, carpal and tarsal hyperextension; when chronic: spontaneous fractures, limb deviations, anorexia, dehydration, loose teeth; when acute: tetany
Phosphorus	%	0.2†-0.6	Generally caused by excessive calcium supplementation. Causes depraved appetite and same signs as a calcium deficiency
Potassium	%	0.4	Caused by excess losses from diarrhea or diuretics, or inadequate intake because of anorexia; causes anorexia, weakness, lethargy, and decreased muscle tone, which may cause head drooping, ataxia, and ascending paralysis

Sodium	%	0.1-0.5‡	Polyuria, salt hunger, pica, weight loss, fatigue, agalactia, and slow growth§
Magnesium	%	0.05-0.10‡	Retarded growth, spreading of toes, hyperextension of carpus and tarsus hyperirritability, convulsions, soft tissue calcification, enlargement of the metaphysis of long bones§
Iron	mg/kg	60	May occur if fed milk exclusively for an extended period or secondary to blood loss; causes microcytic-hypochromic anemia, anisocytosis, and poikilocystosis of erythrocytes
Zinc	mg/kg	50	Anorexia, weight loss, slow growth, emesis, generalized thinning of hair coat, scaly dermatitis, parakeratosis, hair depigmentation, decreased testicular development and wound healing, depression, and peripheral lymphadenopathy
Copper	mg/kg	7	May be caused by excess zinc, iron, or molybdenum; slow growth, bone lesions similar to calcium deficiency, pica, and liver copper less than 20 g/g wet weight. Reported that anemia, hair depigmentation, and diarrhea do not occur in cats as they do in other species
Manganese	mg/kg	5	Impaired reproduction, abortion, enlarged joints, stiffness, reluctance to move; short, thick, and brittle bones§
Iodine	mg/kg	1.5	Hypothyroidism, goiter, alopecia, fetal resorption, cretinism, myxedema, lethargy, drowsiness, timidity; at necropsy, feline thyroid weight >12 mg/100 g body weight

Selenium	mg/kg	0.1	"White muscle disease," skeletal and cardiac myopathy

Table 13: Mineral requirements for dogs and cats and the adverse effects of deficiency. Adapted from a table published in "Complementary and Alternative Veterinary Medicine, Principles and Practice," pp 32-33, edited by A. Schoen and S. Wynn, Mosby, Times Mirror Publications, St. Louis, Missouri, 1998; (permission applied)

*Based on a diet providing 4.0 kcal metabolizable energy/g. For diets with a different caloric density, multiply the amount given times the quotient of (kcal/g of that diet ÷ 4).
†Ca should equal or exceed P, and twice these amounts are recommended during growth and lactation.
‡The greater amount is recommended during lactation.
§This mineral imbalance is rare in dogs and cats.

Several testimonials have been published on the benefits of coral calcium use in dogs, cats and horses. One must be wary of accepting anecdotal reports of health benefit as proof of outcome, but the number of testimonials is becoming impressive as people report improved energy and well-being in pets together with even reports of improvement in bone and joint health (hip dysplasia and simple arthritis) and other beneficial health outcomes. Clearly, coral calcium is playing a role as a newfound holistic supplement for beloved pets. It is interesting to note that folklore in Okinawa described well-being among domestic animals when coral calcium was added to their diet. Scientists at Marine Bio Co. Ltd. have commented on the improved health status of farm animals fed coral calcium supplements but their studies have not been made in a controlled manner. Coral calcium is emerging as a valuable holistic mineral food supplement for dogs, cats and horses.

CHAPTER SUMMARY

The "science" of coral calcium is emerging. The idea that mineral supplements may promote health and wellbeing is not a new notion. Emerging science on the effects of coral calcium on humans is quite fascinating but the information is far from definitive, complete or conclusive. Predictably, the calcium content of coral calcium may be beneficial for bone health (osteoporosis management). Pet owners appear to have discovered potential health benefits of coral calcium in pets. (www.coralcalciumforpets.com) Much more research is required.

**CORAL CALCIUM IS EMERGING
AS A USEFUL MINERAL SUPPLEMENT
FOR DOS, CATS AND HORSES**

CHAPTER 7:

RHETORIC AND FACTOIDS ON CORAL CALCIUM

MORE RHETORIC ABOUT MISGUIDED THOUGHTS ON CORAL CALCIUM

Legal and public objections have been raised about the inappropriate treatment claims made about coral calcium on TV infomercials. Even though future research may demonstrate some of the predicted benefits of the dietary supplement coral calcium, it is wrong to accept potentially false promises of cures with coral calcium. Furthermore, absurd claims about coral calcium will serve to result in premature rejection of the value of coral calcium and provide a disincentive for further research. This situation may be already happening. I have not been able to find any scholarly, "up-to-date account" of the clinical benefits of coral calcium, except to state that the work of Bruce Halstead MD, published in the book, *Fossil Stony Coral Minerals and Their Nutritional Application* (www.wellnesspublishing.com) is worthy of considerable attention.

Conversely, the book, *The Calcium Factor*, self-published by Mr. Robert Barefoot, and bearing the name of the deceased physician, Carl Reich MD, cannot be considered to have substantial content on the subject of coral calcium. In fact, legal disputes exist between Mr. Barefoot and the corporations that own the copyright of the popular book entitled, *Barefoot on Coral Calcium: An Elixir of Life* (www.wellnesspublishing.com). B. Owen D.Ed., author of *Why Calcium?* (Health Digest Books, Cannon Beach, Oregon, 1996) addresses the benefits of coral calcium-treated water. Dr.

Owen has copies of much of the written work of the late Dr. Carl Reich, who is alleged by Mr. Barefoot to have been his principle scientific collaborator. However, Dr. B. Owen has found no evidence of the mention of coral calcium in the work of Dr. Carl Reich who proposed "the calcium deficiency syndrome" as a disease concept. This concept resulted in a style of clinical practice which led to the revocation of Dr. Reich's medical license.

There is more that is unknown about the biological actions of coral calcium than is known. Unfortunately, legal disputes, largely surrounding commercial interests, have overshadowed the public's understanding of coral calcium—these issues cloak the research, development and sale of coral calcium. There are many lessons to be learned from the current disputes which continue to downstage the further study of coral calcium. This nutraceutical is starting to show promise as a unique holistic mineral supplement with uncertain, but fascinating putative benefits in emerging science.

Steeped in folklore, arguments, rhetoric and emerging science, coral calcium is playing an increasing role in America's wide array of putative, health-giving dietary supplements. In fact, coral calcium from Okinawa, Japan has become one of the most popular dietary supplements in the US. *"Response"*, the principal magazine that reports direct marketing results from TV infomercials, shows that TV infomercials on coral calcium enjoyed the number-one ranking of all extended advertising on cable TV for 42 consecutive weeks up to December 2002.

The market response to coral calcium has been frenetic and many health care consumers have questioned their physicians and healthcare-givers about the clinical effects and benefits of this dietary supplement. Unfortunately, consumer confusion about this dietary supplement prevails and clarification about its source, properties and potential biological effects is required. Misunderstandings compound among patients as "marketing hype" and comparison of emerging products, in terms of their advantages or disadvantages, real or imagined, mislead the general public.

Undeniably, marketing predators have purveyed potentially false hope of "cures" with coral calcium to desperate individuals with neurological disability and cancer. Coral calcium is a very interesting holistic source of minerals, principally calcium and magnesium, which runs the risk of being rejected as a useful tool in alternative medicine, as a consequence of zealous and avaricious pro-motion. A number of companies have disavowed themselves of this kind of unethical sales activity (www.naturesbenefit.com).

There is no doubt that coral calcium is a versatile and potent dietary supplement. Coral calcium has attracted considerable re-order business in supplement sales, presumably as a consequence of beneficial effects experienced by consumers of this supplement. Much coral calcium has been sold by TV infomercials that advise, inappropriately, that consumers do not buy coral supplements from responsible sales outlets. Unfortunately, TV sales have not even resulted in consistent distribution of the type of coral calcium dis-cussed on the TV commercials.

The best source of coral calcium is undoubtedly a point of purchase where the seller has an informed opinion about the dif-ferent types of coral calcium and their putative uses. Inappropriate sales and marketing practices have bred rhetoric and arguments that inevitably beleaguer the integrity of the alternative and com-plementary medicine movement.

MARKETING HYPE HURTS
THE ALTERNATIVE MEDICINE MOVEMENT

Our cherished interests in remedies of natural origin are challenged when propaganda and inappropriate treatment claims are made. In many respects, we face a deja-vu in some categories of dietary supplements when marketing hype transcends any rea-sonable level of scientific knowledge or even common sense. For example, shark cartilage was promoted in the 1990's in an illegal manner as a cure for cancer without an adequate basis for a treat-ment claim. **Current circumstances with coral calcium share simi-larities with the saga of shark cartilage.**

Marketing advocates of shark cartilage who made cancer treatment claims have faced ongoing sanctions (more than five years) from the Federal Government. This is an example where the alternative medicine movement must consider the possibility of self-policing. Whereas the involvement of the Federal Government or other regulatory agencies in the growth of natural medicine is often not welcomed, it is now time to examine the source of marketing information about remedies of natural origin. Natural "medicines" do have a useful role in promoting health and well being. Strange as it may seem, extracts of shark cartilage are emerging with new-found promise in cancer research, but earlier hype deflected attention from the research and development of shark cartilage.

Coral calcium may face the same fate as shark cartilage and other dietary supplements that have attracted regulatory discipline, if promoters continue to make unsubstantiated treatment claims. In fact, some of the claims made about the clinical benefits of coral calcium are preposterous: these claims include "grow a new brain," "throw away wheelchairs" and "cure cancer". I trust that readers can recognize the absurd nature of such claims, but there are a substantial number of desperate people who may believe or want to believe in these aphorisms.

PROPAGATION OF MISINFORMATION

Dr. Stephen Barrett, MD, is to be highly commended for his recent investigations of what has been termed "coral calcium scams", in a seven page review of the background of the marketing and misinformation that has been propagated on the subject of coral calcium. I highly recommend that readers ignore silly propoganda. Dr. Barrett has taken some of the claims made by Robert Barefoot and commented on their validity. Clearly, there are many false statements made by Mr. Barefoot in his speeches and writings; and Mr. Barefoot appears to have "questionable credentials", according to Dr. Barrett. The addition of cesium to coral calcium is a problem.

In this book, I have warned that opinion can be very harsh when promoters of dietary supplements cross the line with wild and preposterous treatment claims, together with twisted "pseudo-science". It is clear that there are early signs of my prediction that predatory marketing will "turn people off" and encourage them to be highly critical. However, I do believe that coral calcium is a very interesting dietary supplement with several putative health benefits and it is a very interesting, natural holistic source of minerals. I believe that premature rejection of coral calcium as a valuable dietary supplement is quite unjustified, especially in view of the interesting emerging science with coral calcium supplements in the diet.

OTTO HEINRICH WARBURG BECOMES WIDELY MISQUOTED AND MISREPRESENTED

I never ceased to be amazed by certain individuals who market dietary supplements by twisting good science and using such misinformation to sell products by misrepresentation. Furthermore, I am even more amazed that such marketing predators are so widely believed, even by some practitioners of medicine. In brief, www.encyclopedia.com describes Otto Heinrich Warburg in the following manner *"1883-1970, German physiologist. He was director (1931-53) of the Kaiser Wilhelm Institute (now Max Planck Institute) for cell physiology at Berlin. He investigated the metabolism of tumors and the respiration of cells, particularly cancer cells. For his discovery of the nature and the mode of action of (Warburg's) yellow enzyme, he won the 1931 Nobel Prize in Physiology or Medicine. He edited The Metabolism of Tumors (tr. 1931) and wrote New Methods of Cell Physiology (1962)."*

Tracing Dr. Otto Warburg's work does lead to a conclusion that he was convinced that cancerous cells could live and develop in the absence of oxygen. However, Dr. Warburg's theories have been rejected as "old hat" by many distinguished cancer researchers. Mr. Robert Barefoot has misquoted the work of Otto Warburg in support of his notions of body oxygenation with calcium - an absurd proposal. The cherished and important work of Dr. Warburg should not be contaminated by this kind of pseudo-science. Much information on Otto Heinrich Warburg, a Nobel Prize winner is to be found in the book entitled "The Warburgs", Ron Chermow, Random House, 1993. This book also discusses the life of Eric Warburg, a distant relative of Otto Warburg who was Hitler's authority on cancer and who enjoyed a special protected status during the reign of The Third Reich in Germany. One very strange website describes associations between Dr. Reich, the alleged co-author of the book "The Calcium Factor" that is touted by Robert Barefoot. This website (www.stopcancer.com) states "Robert Barefoot being a biochemist such as Otto Warburg has enough knowledge to put the remaining pieces together" – referring to the inaccurate self-published books "The Calcium Factor" and "Death by Diet". This is patent nonsense and, upon information and belief, Mr. Barefoot is not a biochemist and he has no formal biomedical training.

There are so many inaccuracies and misstatements about coral calcium and its health benefits that it would be possible to write a book on the misinformation. For example, Mr. Barefoot discusses the enhanced oxygenation of tissues when blood pH is alkaline. In fact, exactly the reverse is sometimes true. Hemoglobin will donate more oxygen to tissues in the presence of blood acidity which favors oxygen dissociation from hemoglobin. This knowledge of basic physiology seems to be mysterious to Mr. Barefoot and many other people who believe him.

FACTOIDS

Many consumers of coral calcium are confused by inaccurate statements about the composition and potential biological actions of coral calcium (marine coral minerals or fossilized stony coral minerals). The following facts and conclusions from available information may help dispel some of the marketing "mumbo-jumbo" on coral calcium:

1) Testimonials of the benefits of coral calcium are not proof of a consistent, beneficial health effect. However, the volume of testimonials of benefits cannot be ignored and should be further explored. The continuing use of coral calcium by many people as a consequence of their perceived benefit is an important issue.

2) Calcium contained in coral calcium is not 100% absorbed, nor is it completely ionized in the human gastrointestinal tract in most people.

3) Coral calcium supplements do not contain "microbes." They are treated in a manner that eliminates bacteria, fungi, molds and other living material. Marine "microbes" are not probiotic agents with beneficial effects on the human gastrointestinal tract.

4) While the magnesium content of coral collected below sea level may be higher than coral collected above sea level, a consistent balance of calcium to magnesium of 2:1 probably does not occur in nature in the coral sand precursor of the dietary supplement coral calcium. Below sea-collected

coral is blended probably to bring up the magnesium content to 12%, approximately. I use the word "probably" with caution; arguments prevail in the dietary supplement industry.

5) There is no clear evidence whatsoever to state that below-sea-collected coral sand results in a more effective coral calcium supplement than land-collected (mined) coral sand. Some evidence suggests that above-sea level collected coral calcium is more suitable for use as a supplement, at least in terms of both safety, efficacy and ecological appropriateness. These matters remain unresolved.

6) Statements that coral calcium cures or prevents cancer are not scientific facts. The media statements that individuals can "grow new brains" or cure degenerative neurological illness, such as Parkinson's disease, are absurd remarks. The individuals purveying false hope to people with tragic illness must be sanctioned. These acts are despicable.

7) Coral calcium probably works by mechanisms other than its content of calcium alone (see Dr. Bruce Halstead's work).

8) Mr. Robert Barefoot, author of *Barefoot on Coral Calcium: An Elixir of Life*, is not a medical practitioner or experienced biomedical scientist, according to reports. He is a chemist who worked in the petroleum industry. Bruce Halstead MD was a highly experienced, marine biologist, medical doctor and expert in the health applications of marine products or materials. He has written one of the most valuable, extensive documents on marine toxicology that has been used by several governments. Dr. Halstead believed that only above sea-collected (land) coral should be used for coral calcium supplements (see the book, *Fossilized Stony Coral Minerals and their Nutritional Application*, by B. Halstead MD).

9) Several companies <u>claim</u> that Mr. Robert Barefoot has donated his likeness (sometimes on an exclusive basis) to sell coral calcium supplements. Mr. Barefoot has variably promoted and endorsed the use of coral calcium in all forms: above-ground collected, below-sea collected and teabag-enclosed coral to make coral water. Currently, he seems to favor below-sea collected coral. Several disputes have arisen over the use of Mr. Barefoot's likeness, especially in relation

to TV commercials.

10) The use of coral calcium should be guided by fact, not speculation. Much about the benefits, or lack thereof, of coral calcium remains unknown. The use of coral calcium should not be guided entirely by a likeness, personality or endorsement.

11) At the time of this writing, the only company that provides both forms of coral (above- and below-sea-collected coral sand) in four clearly labeled products is Natures Benefit Inc. and specifications of these products are published on the Internet at www.naturesbenefit.com and www.coralcalciuminformation.com.

12) Books written on the subject of coral calcium are not to be confused as labels on products. They represent only authors' opinions (including this book!).

13) Testimonials in the use of coral calcium do not often define the type of coral calcium used e.g. by brand, by type, by delivery (above-sea or below-sea collected in capsules or enclosed in tea bags). Some coral calcium is cut with "fillers", e.g. chalk.

14) Much misleading information exists on the Internet and in books written on the subject of coral calcium. Many Internet sites promise cures of diseases with coral calcium and while these alleged "cures" may have appeared in testimonials, there are no controlled clinical trials on specific disease treatments with coral calcium.

15) Coral calcium is a valuable, natural holistic mineral supplement, containing many potential micronutrients.

16) While magnesium intake is important, calcium and magnesium compete for absorption. This means that magnesium can interfere with calcium absorption and vice versa. The ideal ratio of intake of calcium to magnesium in the human diet is the subject on ongoing debate among scientists.

17) Recommendations for high doses of vitamin D are dangerous and serious toxicity may occur with continued use.

18) No evidence exists to support the use of cesium, nickel or silver as nutritional supplements. These are toxic elements at significant levels of intake or with chronic continued use. Cesium is not a proven cancer cure.

19) Uncontrolled, excessive exposure to sunlight is damaging to health.

20) Dr. Otto Warburg did not have coral calcium in mind when he described his Nobel Prize-winning research; and calcium intake is not a primary way of supplying oxygen to the body. Mr. Barefoot has seriously misinterpreted the work of Dr. Warburg and others.

21) Measurements of the pH of body fluids are not an accurate, reproducible or even useful way of gauging the intake of minerals. Measurements of the pH of saliva for guiding mineral supplement intake are probably valueless. Coral teabags that show rapid shifts in the pH of water towards alkalinity may often contain "baking soda" (sodium bicarbonate) or calcinated coral sand (calcium oxide). The actual contents of some teabags containing coral are not always listed on labels.

22) Coral calcium does not "dissolve" completely in water.

23) The Food and Drug Administration does not condone treatment claims on supplements; those that make such claims are breaking the law.

24) Companies that sell coral calcium with treatment claims must be avoided.

25) Many types of coral calcium are sold. These dietary supplements differ in their manufacture, additives, etc. The term "coral calcium" is not an accurate description of coral minerals used as a dietary supplement. Coral minerals are a source of many minerals, often in small amounts.

26) Mr. Barefoot states "all coral is fantastic." This may not be the case.

27) Bruce Halstead MD believes that the micronutrient (elemental) trace components of coral calcium exert important biological effects. This may or may not be the case.

28) The only significant scientific observations on the use of coral calcium in potential disease management relate to osteoporosis.

29) While the presence of coral calcium in the environment of Okinawa may contribute to longevity, many other factors operate.

30) Many people claim a benefit from taking coral calcium – a

fact. More research is required to assess these reports of benefit.

THE CONSUMERS CHOICE OF CORAL CALCIUM

I have purposely avoided any lengthy discussion of testimonials on the health benefits of coral calcium. Some people argue that these testimonials are proof of benefit, while others demand controlled scientific studies as proof of health benefits. When it comes to choosing a coral calcium supplement, there are several important issues to address.

First, the coral calcium supplement should be clearly labeled and, ideally, the source of coral calcium should be identified, but this has not been consistent in the marketplace. Second, the coral calcium supplement should be of food grade and it should not contain toxic heavy metals or organic pollutants. Third, only forms of coral calcium supplements for which there is a precedent of beneficial use should be used. While these general principles apply without argument, there are at least 100 brands of coral calcium available in the U.S. market, differing in source, dosage, processing and delivery (see www.wellnesspublishing.com and www.naturesbenefit.com).

In conclusion, the mechanism of action of coral calcium as a health-promoting supplement remains in doubt. High-quality coral calcium fossils collected from below or above sea level appear to have equivalent reported health benefits (anecdotal), but more studies are required. That said, the perceived benefits reported by the thousands of people taking coral calcium supplements cannot be ignored. Consumers must be given a choice of high-grade coral supplements, but more important, they must be given accurate information in order to make an informed choice (www.naturesbenefit.com, www.coralcalciummagazine.com, www.coralcalciuminformation.com). **What is most impressive is the continuity of use of this mineral supplement by many consumers, which has occurred largely as a consequence of benefits experienced.** Coral calcium is here to stay as an under-explored, valuable dietary supplement that must not be misunderstood.

AFTERWORD

Steeped in folklore, arguments, rhetoric and emerging science, coral calcium is playing an increasing role in America's wide array of putative, health-giving food supplements. In fact, coral calcium from Okinawa, Japan has become one of the most popular dietary supplements in the U.S. Consumer confusion about this dietary supplement prevails and clarification about its source, properties and potential biological effects is required. This book was revised into its second edition in March 2003 because of mounting public confusion about the use of coral calcium as a dietary supplement.

The development of interest in coral calcium as a food supplement reminds one of other phases in the popularization of some nutraceuticals where hype may have transcended science. This circumstance tends to threaten any valuable category of dietary supplement. A dietary supplement can become damaged by excessive promotion and the propagation of misleading information. In contrast to statements in the preface of the first edition of this book, I believe that some individuals have given intentionally misleading information on the subject of coral calcium. Furthermore, some purveyors of coral calcium have made wild treatment claims that can only serve to damage this valuable category of mineral supplements. The enthusiasm for promoting a dietary supplement sometimes overtakes hard facts. This has happened and continues to happen with many classes of dietary supplements, much to the detriment of the nutraceutical industry.

In this second edition of *Natures Benefit from Coral Calcium*, I try to educate myself and others on the science of remedies of natural origin. I am not a self-proclaimed expert on coral calcium. Furthermore, I do not know all the answers to questions posed on the subject of coral calcium; and I must make it clear that my interest in coral calcium as a supplement was fuelled more than 10 years ago from an initial position of skepticism. My interest in coral calcium has graduated to the point of belief in this dietary supplement as potentially powerful, poorly understood, promoter of health and well-being. In this book, I explore how and why coral calcium could work to benefit health, but I can only speculate on its potential biopharmaceutical actions. However, I can sort some facts from the many silly speculations about this valuable nutraceutical.

There is no doubt that the interest in coral calcium has swept the nation. From humble beginnings as a means of purifying water, coral calcium has been promoted in network marketing, radio shows, books, articles and more recently, national TV infomercials. In the dietary supplement industry, one witnesses a repetitive phenomenon with product promotions, where the use of the supplement is driven more by the charisma and personality of the promoters, than it is by the clinical science behind the product. **I stress that we have little in the way of controlled clinical studies on the benefits of coral calcium, but there may be thousands of testimonials concerning its benefit.** The research that is available on coral calcium is reported in this book. Scientific studies on the subject remain relatively scant, but initial outcomes seem promising.

Marine biologists have clarified much about the habitat and composition of live coral and its fossilized remnants, mixed with biogenous sediments, which have been called "coral calcium." This book attempts to sort out science (or facts) from speculation on the subject of the source and processing of coral calcium from Okinawa, Japan. The many anecdotal reports of the benefits of coral calcium are screaming to be further explored in scientific studies. However, much uninformed rhetoric about its origins, characteristics and biomedical applications must be questioned. I have committed myself over the past three years to examine the origin, quality and biological characteristics of coral calcium in order that people may make informed judgments about its use and potential benefit. While I repeat that I am not a self-proclaimed expert on the subject of coral calcium, I am a student of its promise for supporting health and well being. My curiosity in alternative medicine has been present for 30 years and it has dominated my thoughts for 10 years.

There is a risk, as my publishers keep telling me, of writing books that nobody wants to read. There is more than a measure of truth in the statement that "the truth hurts". This reasoning should not apply to our quest for knowledge about the benefits of remedies of natural origin. Without open dialogue and rational arguments, there will be no material advances in natural medicines. **Nutritional medicine has attracted more than its fair share of wishful thinkers.** While such people sell products, they damage the general perception about remedies of natural origin.

APPENDIX

ANALYSIS OF CORAL CALCIUM SAMPLES

This section is a technical review of research to date on the physical and chemical characteristics of coral calcium.

There has been no published study of the physical characteristics of coral calcium, as they relate to different forms of coral calcium that may be used in dietary supplements. Unpublished observations of the electron microscopic appearance of coral calcium have been presented (Holt S, "Coral Calcium Clarifications," presented at Western Expo, Anaheim CA, March 2003). These high-powered microscopic studies of coral calcium have shown evidence of porosity (see Chapter 1, Figures 1A and 1B). The purveyors of dietary supplements have a responsibility to research the physico-chemical characteristics of materials used in supplements, but few manufacturers have accepted this responsibility. I have collaborated with Andy Bowers of Coral, Inc. and Dr. Sam Iyengar, Ph.D. on the characterization of different types of coral calcium material using a variety of standard, but relatively complex, scientific methods. I report a very preliminary set of data on the analysis of different types of coral calcium samples and the results are fascinating and quite illuminating. However, I stress that the research is incomplete and it cannot be subject to premature judgment.

In recent studies, sponsored by Coral, Inc. of Nevada, three samples of coral calcium were analyzed using techniques of x-ray diffraction, x-ray crystallography, energy dispersive x-ray analysis, scanning electron microscopy and thermogravimetric studies. These techniques permit the study of the structure (morphology), mineralogical (mineral content) and chemical composition of coral calcium samples. The three samples of coral calcium powder used in the studies were: 1. marine coral calcium "low Mg", collected below sea level in Okinawa, Japan, 2. marine coral calcium "high Mg", collected below sea level in Okinawa, Japan, and 3. land coral calcium collected above sea level, with its typical low magnesium content.

Sample 1, the "low magnesium," below-sea coral calcium, showed evidence of a primary content of calcite ($CaCO_3$) with magnesium substitution within the calcite. In addition, the sample contained aragonite. Aragonite is a calcium containing mineral that is relatively unstable, but typical of natural (organic) sources of minerals. In addition, scanning electron microscopy revealed porosity of the particles in this form of coral calcium (below sea, low magnesium). These findings contrast the observations in sample 3 (land coral). In the land coral, well formed crystals of calcite appear without notable amounts of magnesium incorporation. Again, porosity is apparent in the particles in the land coral.

Most striking were the findings in the second sample which was coral calcium collected below sea level with a "high magnesium" content. This is the type of coral that is advertised and sold as naturally balanced coral calcium with a ratio of calcium to magnesium of 2:1. In some circumstances, this has been described, arguably, as the "highest grade of coral," a statement that is not supported by any known or proven advantage of this form of coral in terms of biological functions or efficacy as a supplement. Certainly, this form of coral is generally more expensive to purchase than the other two types of coral.

Careful studies using the techniques of physico-chemical analyses described earlier showed that this high-magnesium containing, below-sea collected coral, contained mostly dolomite ($CaMg(CO_3)_2$). Furthermore, scanning electron micrographs (high-powered microscopic pictures) showed well developed crystals in this sample of high magnesium containing coral calcium and energy dispersive x-ray analysis (EDS) confirmed significant amounts of magnesium in the sample.

The study results on the high magnesium containing marine coral imply clearly that this material is predominantly dolomite. The nature of dolomite requires some explanation. The word dolomite is derived from the name of an 18th century French geologist (Dolomieu). In essence, dolomite is rock consisting mainly of calcium carbonate and magnesium carbonate and it is basically "lime-stone" or "marble" with significant magnesium carbonate present. The mineralogical studies to date could be interpreted that the high magnesium containing below-sea collected coral calcium is, per-haps, more removed in origin from live coral than is coral calcium collected from land masses or from regular ocean floor collections, where low magnesium containing coral sand is collected as a pre-cursor to this dietary supplement coral calcium. This is arguable.

Recent studies involving thermogravimetric analysis of coral calcium reveals interesting preliminary results. In the process of thermogravimetric analysis, the samples are heated to very high temperatures (up to 1,000 degrees Centigrade). The liberation of water during heating causes weight change in the samples and CO_2 is lost during heating by disruption of the carbonate portion of the coral calcium. Dr. Iyengar, Ph.D., an expert in mineralogical analy-ses and material sciences, studied a branch from a whole sample of dead coral (coral was an intact sample; data on file Coral, Inc., Nevada). Powder prepared from the branch of coral and other coral calcium samples (referred to above) were heated. Significant weight loss occurred at lower temperatures (300-400 degrees Centigrade, approximately) in the sample of coral material taken from the coral branch than in the coral calcium samples whereas loss of weight in the other coral calcium samples became significant above the tem-perature of 800 degrees Centigrade, approximately. These findings imply that perhaps there is more organic material retained in intact branches of dead coral compared with coral calcium supplements which are derived from coral sand precursors. In simple terms, intact coral branches, or lumps of dead coral, may contain more organic matter, e.g. dead carboniferous material (dead "organisms" or "plants"?).

Biochemical (biogenous) sediment in sea water is derived from marine life that has extracted dissolved mineral matter, such as calcite and silica to form shells or other hard parts of living marine life, such as the stony-house of coral polyps. This material collects in quantities at the ocean bottom around the island chains of Okinawa and forms raw material for the creation of some sedi-mentary rocks that lie on the ocean floor. A good example of this type of activity is found in the south of England, where the white chalk cliffs of Dover are composed of limestone that have been lithified (formed into a rock) and lifted above sea level (compare with Okinawa, Japan). The most common type of sedimentary rock that is formed from distant biogenous sediments is calcite-rich limestone. Indeed, any close examination of limestone adjacent to seashores reveals marine-derived fragments, such as shells, within the body of the rocks.

Oceanographic studies have shown that "subduction zones" on the floor of the ocean can form around island chains. Examples of subduction zones are to be found in regions southwest of Alaska and around the islands of Okinawa in southern Japan. There are platforms of older rocks exposed above sea level in this process of subduction that involves past activity of volcanoes. This older type of rock underlies many islands throughout the world but it is often submerged and is not able to be directly observed in the same way that it can be spotted in certain locations, such as the islands of Okinawa, Japan. We have learned that marine organisms, such as coral polyps, and algae form calcareous deposits which can produce a thick layer of calcareous (calcium containing) material on the ocean floor around the Ryukyus Islands. The jigsaw puzzle is now starting to fit together, but some of the pieces are missing!

Examining the formation of the stony-house of live coral gives insight into how the remnants of these marine organisms ultimately form the interesting geological findings in Okinawa. A coral reef is the sum total of the net accumulation of calcium carbonate with other minerals, most notably magnesium within the living infrastructure of the coral reef. Calcium carbonate tends to harden with the application of gravity of 2.6 g/cm?, and high temperature accelerates hardening (volcanoes?).

Minerals found commonly in samples of coral reefs include aragonite ($CaCO_3$), calcite ($CaCO_3$) and Mg-substituted calcite. Aragonites are not very stable at atmospheric temperatures and pressures. In brief, the remnants of the coral reef may ultimately form dolomite, presumably at deep locations in the ocean where higher gravitational pressures exist and variable thermal changes could have occurred from volcanic activity. In summary, it could be reasonably concluded that high magnesium containing coral sand collected from the ocean floor around the Ryukyus Islands is not as closely related to live coral exoskeletons, as are other forms of coral sands?

One can see just how complex arguments may become as we further identify the physical and chemical characteristic of substances that are sold under the name coral calcium in dietary supplements. The findings that I describe support my earlier conclusions that one must not be quick to accept speculations about different types of coral calcium, in terms of their "grade" or "quality". What may be described as the "highest" grade may not be the "highest" grade and grading coral calcium is a complex issue for scientists to examine.

Perhaps more important than the described basic science observations are the clinical outcomes that are obtained with different types of coral calcium used as dietary supplements. Unfortunately, the claims of benefit surrounding the use of coral calcium do not define the type of coral calcium used and there is no doubt that many testimonials support both the use of land coral calcium or below-sea coral calcium; and even the drinking of coral mineral-enriched water. Much more basic science research is required, and marketing people who talk generally about different grades or quality of coral, clearly, do not understand the science required to adopt an opinion of value.

REFERENCES

Asai K, *Miracle Cure*. Organic germanium, Japan Publications, Tokyo – cited by B. Halstead MD.

Barefoot R, *Barefoot on Coral Calcium: An Elixir of Life*, Wellness Publishing, www.wellnesspublishing.com, 2001.

Bianchi CF, *Cell Calcium*. Appleton – Century Crofts, London, 1968.

Boericke OE, Boericke Pocket *Manual of Homeopathic Material Medica with Repertory*, B. Jain Publishers Letd. New Delhi, 1992 (reprint edition).

Curtin ME, *Chemicals from the Sea*, Biotechnology, 3, 1, 34, 36-37, 1985.

Der Marderosian A, Liberti L, *Natural Product Medicine*, George F. Stickley Co, PA, 1988.

Farish DJ, *Human Biology*, Jones and Bartlett Publishers, Boston, 1975.

Faulkner DJ, *Marine Natural Products, Natural Product Reports*, 3, 1, 1-33, 1986.

Faulkner D, Chesher R, *Living Corals*, CN Potter Inc., NY, 1979.

Grant Gross M, *Oceanography, A View of the Earth*, Prentice-Hall Inc, NJ, 1977.

Halstead BW and CL Foster, *Drugs from the Sea, Chinese J. Mar. Drugs*, 9(1):1-32, 1990.

Halstead BW and TC Rozema, *The Scientific Basis of EDTA Chelation Therapy*, TRC Publishing, Landrum, SC, 1997.

Halstead BW, *Fossil Stony Coral Minerals and Their Nutritional Application*, Health Digest Publishing Company, Cannon Beach, Oregon, 1999.

Halstead BW, *Poisonous and Venomous Marine Animals of the World*, The Darwin Press Inc., Princeton, NJ, 1988.

Halstead BW, *The Scientific Basis of EDTA Chelation Therapy*, Golden Quill Press, Colton, CA, 1979.

Holliday L, Wood E, *Coral Reefs*, Salamander Books, New York, 1989.

Holt S, Bader D, *Natures Benefit for Pets*, Wellness Publishing.

Holt S, Barilla J, *The Power of Cartilage*, Kensington Publishers, NY, 1998.

Holt S, Comac L, *Miracle Herbs*, Carol Publishing, NJ, 1997.

Holt S, *Natural Ways to Digestive Health*, M. Evans Inc., NY, NY, 2000.

Holt S, *The Natural Way to a Healthy Heart*, M. Evans Inc., NY, NY, 1999.

Holt S, *The Soy Revolution*, Dell Publishing, Random House, NY, NY, 1999.

Kent JT, *Repertory of the Homeopathic Materia Medica with Word Index*, B. Jain Publishers Ltd, New Delhi, 1991.

Kobyashi J, *The Secret of Health and Longevity in Okinawa*, *The Sokai*, Okinawa, 1990 – cited by B. W. Halstead.

Lindlahr H, *Natural Therapeutics, Vol III, Dietetics*, Edited by Proby J, C.W. Daniel Company Ltd, Walden, UK, 1914, revised in 1983.

Lindlahr H, *Philosophy of Natural Therapeutics*, C.W. Daniel Company Ltd, 1914, revisions and additions by J. Proby, 1975, reprinted 1993.

NIH, *Optimal Calcium Intake*, National Institutes of Health, 12, 4, 1-24, 1994.

Rolfe L, Lennon N, *Nature's 12 Magic Healers: The Amazing Secrets of Cell Salts*, Parker Publishing Company, Inc., West Nyack, NY, 1978.

Scheuer P, *Chemistry of Marine Natural Products*, Academic Press, NY, 1973.

Tarbuck EJ, *Earth Science*, Charles E. Merrill Publishing Company, Columbus, 1979, pp. 229-233.

Ullman D, *Discovering Homeopathy*, North Atlantic Books, Berkely, CA, 1991.

Walford RL, *The 120 Year Diet, How to Double Your Vital Years*, Simon and Schuster, NY, 1986.

Willcox BJ, Willcox DC, Makoto Suzuki, *The Okinawa Program: How the world's longest-lived people achieve everlasting health – and how you can too*, Clarkson Potter/Publishers, NY, NY, 2000.

WEB SITES

www.wellnesspublishing.com, *books on coral calcium.*

www.naturesbenefit.com, *commercial sources of coral calcium.*

www.coralcalciuminformation.com, *up-to-date information.*

www.antiporosis.com, *commercial information on coral calcium for bone health*

www.calciodecoral.net, *commercial information in Spanish.*

www.antiagingmethods.com, *prevent premature death.*

www.combatsyndromeX.com, *the most important public health initiative.*

www.naturescalcium.com, *eggshell calcium.*

www.coralcalciummagazine.com, *a source of information.*

ABOUT THE AUTHOR

Stephen Holt MD is a board certified gastroenterologist and industry best-selling author from New York. Dr. Holt is a frequent guest lecturer at scientific meetings and a popular media expert on therapeutics. (www.sholtmd.com)

Other books by the author:

Holt S, *The Soy Revolution*, Dell Publishing, Random House, NY, NY, 1999 (third printing 2002).

Holt S, *The Natural Way to a Healthy Heart*, M. Evans Inc., 1999 (second printing 2002).

Holt S, *Natural Ways to Digestive Health*, M. Evans Inc., 2000 (second printing 2002).

Holt S, Comac L, *Miracle Herbs*, Carol Publishing, NJ, 1997.

Holt S, Barilla J, *The Power of Cartilage*, Kensington Publishers, NY, 1998.

Holt S, Bader D, *Natures Benefit For Pets*, Wellness Publishing, 2001.

Holt S, *Natures Benefit From Coral Calcium: Sorting Science from Speculation*, Wellness Publishing, 2002.

Holt S, *The Antiporosis Plan*, Wellness Publishing, 2002

Holt S, *Combat Syndrome X, Y and Z*, Wellness Publishing, 2002

Holt S, *Natures Sleep*, Wellness Publishing, 2003 (in press)

Holt S, *Digestion*, www.naturaldigestion.com, 2003 (in press)

Dr. Holt's books are available in major bookstores and on the Internet at www.wellnesspublishing.com.

NATURES BENEFIT, INC.

The Leader in Coral Calcium

presents

CORAL CALCIUM
from
OKINAWA, JAPAN

The Marine Miracle© Available in FOUR Forms:

- **Barefoot Coral Calcium Plus™**
  PURE CORAL with Added Vital Nutrients

- **Halstead Stony Coral Minerals
  Coral Calcium™**

- **Marine Coral Minerals™**
  100% Pure, High Quality Coral
  with balanced magnesium.

- **Coral Calcium Powder™**

**www.naturesbenefit.com
Telephone: 1-888-765-1099**

ACCEPT NO OTHER BRAND©
High Grade Coral from Okinawa, Japan

CORAL CALCIUM
IS AVAILABLE IN
FOUR FORMS:

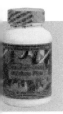

· Barefoot Coral Calcium Plus™ is high grade below sea collected coral with a 2:1 balance of calcium to magnesium. It has added vitamins and nutrients.

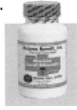

· Marine Coral Minerals™ is high quality pure coral calcium with magnesium collected below sea level, and balanced 2:1 calcium to magnesium.

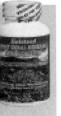

· Halstead Stony Coral Minerals Coral Calcium™ is a high quality pure coral calcium from land deposits of coral remnants.

· Coral Calcium Powder™ is 100% pure coral collected from land deposits in Okinawa, Japan.

• Coral Calcium is more than a calcium supplement. It is a holistic mixture of minerals derived from coral remnants. It is collected from deposits around coral reefs below sea level, or from the land in Okinawa, Japan.

• Live coral is not harmed during collection of Coral Calcium. It is the parts of the reef that are dropped in the ocean from wave action and other natural occurences that form coral calcium.

• Natures Benefit Inc. uses only the highest grade coral containing different types of trace minerals or micronutrients. Natures Benefit, Inc. uses two types of Coral in it's four Coral Calcium products.

Detailed product specifications are shown at www.naturesbenefit.com

Coral Calcium Information Center
Email: info@naturesbenefit.com
or Fax: 973-824-8822

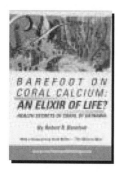

Robert. R Barefoot's
Book on Coral Calcium

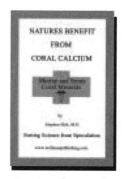

Dr. Stephen Holt's
Book on
Coral Calcium

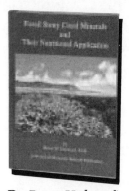

Dr. Bruce Halstead's
Book: Fossil Stony Coral
Minerals and Their
Nutritional Application

Coral Calcium - A Marine Miracle©
The demand for coral calcium from Okinawa, Japan has swept the nation. This supplement is identified as a revolutionary source of minerals. Coral Calcium is a dietary supplement. If ever a product was misnamed, it is "coral calcium", because the contents of this marine miracle are more versatile than calcium alone. Perhaps, this valuable nutritional supplement is best called marine or stony coral minerals.

Information
An information source on coral is available through email at: info@naturesbenefit.com or by fax at 973-824-8822, given the overwhelming request for information by the public. In brief, encapsulated coral is enjoying extreme popularity! Coral can be taken "plain" in capsules such as Marine Coral Minerals™ and Halstead Stony Coral™ or Coral Calcium Powder™, or with added nutrients (eg: vitamins D & E) such as found in capsule formulas discussed and recommended by Robert R. Barefoot.

The History of Coral Calcium Use
Japanese folklore and contemporary scientific opinion indicates that coral calcium has nutritional benefits. The most informative source of information on the health benefits of coral calcium is to be found in the books displayed at www.wellnesspublishing.com. These books discuss the colorful folklore history behind coral including the belief that the consumption of marine coral supports health and longevity. The citizens of Okinawa, Japan often live to a ripe old age in good health. Testimonials on the beneficial use of coral calcium as a dietary supplement are measured in thousands and are astonishing, according to Mr. Barefoot, whose work has been commended by contemporary nutritionists, including G. Scott Miller, known in health circles as "the Mineral Man".

Note: These books are not dietary supplement labeling

NATURES BENEFIT PET DIVISION PRESENTS: CORAL CALCIUM POWDER FOR PETS™

www.coralcalciumforpets.com

Many people have requested the availability of coral calcium in a convenient form for their beloved companion animals. High-quality coral calcium is available for pets in the new product "Coral Calcium for Pets™." The unique micromineral profile of coral calcium provides calcium co-factors for the chemistry of life (up to 75 trace minerals).
A 90 gram-powder with a scoop that permits graded doses for dogs, cats and horses of different body weights.

To order call 1-888-CORAL-CALCIUM

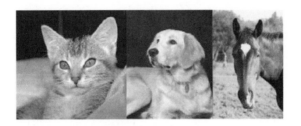

LOVE YOUR PET AND VISIT YOUR VET

Cartivet Plus,
Cartequine Plus,
Suprazyme,
Tranquil,
Proud,
Natural Ear Comfort,
Oral Biocleanse,
The Omega Factor,
Liposome Angio-Inhibitor,

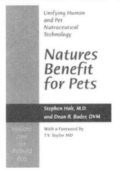

Unifying Human and Pet Nutraceutical Technology

Natures Benefit for Pets

Stephen Holt, M.D. and Dean R. Bader, DVM

With a Foreword by T.V. Taylor MD

ASK ABOUT OUR FREE BOOK OFFER AND COMPLETE LINE OF NATURAL PRODUCTS FOR PETS

The advice of a veterinarian is recommended for pups and kittens.

NOT FOR USE IN EXOTIC PETS.